Getting into

Physiotherapy Courses

James Griffith

11th edition

trotman | t

Getting into guides

Getting into Art & Design Courses, 12th edition
Getting into Business & Economics Courses, 15th edition
Getting into Dental School, 13th edition
Getting into Engineering Courses, 7th edition
Getting into Law, 14th edition
Getting into Medical School 2024 Entry, 28th edition
Getting into Oxford & Cambridge 2024 Entry, 26th edition
Getting into Pharmacy and Pharmacology Courses, 2nd edition
Getting into Psychology Courses, 14th edition
Getting into Veterinary School, 12th edition
How to Complete Your UCAS Application 2024 Entry, 35th edition

Getting into Physiotherapy Courses
This 11th edition published in 2023 by Trotman Education, an imprint of Trotman Indigo Publishing Ltd, 21d Charles Street, Bath BA1 1HX

© Trotman Indigo Publishing Ltd 2023

Author: James Griffith

10th–9th edns: Philip Shanahan
8th–5th edns: James Barton
4th edn: James Burnett
3rd edn: James Burnett & Maya Waterstone
2nd–1st edns: James Burnett & Andrew Long

British Library Cataloguing in Publication Data
A catalogue record for this book is available from the British Library.

ISBN 978 1 912943 54 8

All rights reserved. This book is sold subject to the condition that it shall not, by way of trade or otherwise, be lent, resold, hired out or otherwise circulated without the publisher's prior written consent in any form of binding or cover other than that in which it is published and without a similar condition including this condition being imposed on the subsequent purchaser. No part of this publication may be reproduced, stored in a retrieval system or transmitted in any form or by any means, electronic and mechanical, photocopying, recording or otherwise without prior permission of Trotman Indigo Publishing.

Every effort has been made to trace copyright holders and to obtain their permission for the use of copyright material. The publisher apologises for any errors or omissions and would be grateful to be notified of any corrections that should be incorporated in future editions of this book.

Printed and bound in the UK by Ashford Colour Press Ltd.

Contents

About the author	vi
Acknowledgements	vii
Warming up: Introduction	**1**
What is physiotherapy?	3
What do physiotherapists do?	3
About this book	5
1| Pressure points: Careers	**7**
Working as a physiotherapist	8
Common career paths for physiotherapists	9
Employment prospects	11
Continuing Professional Development	13
Occupational therapy	13
2| Strengthen your core: Physiotherapy courses: what to expect	**17**
Typical course structure	18
Research dissertation	19
Elective clinical placement	19
Teaching styles	19
Courses in Scotland	20
Courses in Wales	22
Courses in Northern Ireland	23
MSc (pre-registration) course	23
3| Pulled in every direction: Work experience	**25**
Length of time	26
How to apply	27
Work experience in Wales	29
Things to look out for during work experience	29
Tips for work experience	31
Discussing your work experience at interview	32
4| On the rack/under observation: The UCAS application	**33**
Choice of university	33
Entrance requirements	35
Your choices	37
The UCAS application form	39
Making your application stand out	40

Contents

	When to submit the UCAS application	42
	Deferred entry	42
	What happens next?	43
5|	**Tweak it: The personal statement**	**45**
	Why physiotherapy?	45
	What have you done to investigate physiotherapy?	46
	Personal qualities	47
	Extracurricular activities	47
	General tips	48
6|	**At full stretch: The interview**	**53**
	Questions to get you relaxed	53
	Questions about physiotherapy	55
	Questions to find out what sort of person you are	58
	How to succeed in your interview	59
	How you are selected	65
7|	**Do you know your gluteus maximus from your articulatio cubiti? Current issues**	**67**
	The NHS Long Term Plan	67
	Concussion	69
	Technology in physiotherapy	71
	Mental Health	73
	An ageing population	73
	Obesity	74
	Parkinson's disease	76
	Repetitive strain injury	77
	Rehabilitation of stroke patients	78
	Exercise referral schemes	79
	Stand up for your health	79
	Physiotherapists given prescribing powers	80
	Brexit and the NHS	81
	Alternative therapies	81
8|	**Massaging the results: Results day**	**83**
	What to do if you have no offer	83
	What to do if you hold an offer but miss the grades	85
	Retaking your A levels	86
9|	**The fifth metatarsal: Non-standard applications**	**89**
	Students who have not studied science A levels	89
	International students	90
	Mature students	91
	Graduates	91
	Applicants with no suitable academic qualifications	91
	Access courses	92

	Physiotherapy degree apprenticeships	92
	Students with disabilities and special educational needs	93
10|	**Make no bones about it: Fees and funding**	**95**
	Fees	95
	Bursaries, sponsorship and grants	96
	Work while you study	97
11|	**Exercise the mind: Useful information and further resources**	**99**
	Universities offering physiotherapy degrees	99
	Useful resources	103
	Other useful addresses	104
	Useful websites	105
	Further reading	106
12|	**Don't be bone idle: Glossary**	**107**
	Postscript	**109**
	Notes	**110**

About the author

James Griffith is a Director of Recruitment for the Mander Portman Woodward college group. James works within the International team, leading on student recruitment predominantly from Africa, the Middle East, Europe and the Commonwealth of Independent States (CIS). As part of this role, James interviews students as part of their admissions process to MPW, offering advice on the right study path to take for their dream university and course.

Acknowledgements

Many thanks are due to all those who have written previous editions of *Getting into Physiotherapy Courses*, including Philip Shanahan, James Burnett, Maya Waterstone, Andrew Long and James Barton.

I would also like to especially thank the Chartered Society of Physiotherapy for the huge amount of information they provided for the completion of this book.

The information in this book has come from a variety of sources and is, I believe, correct at the time of going to press. However, the views expressed are my own and any errors are down to me.

I hope that you find this book a valuable and helpful source, and I wish you all the success in your future endeavours in physiotherapy.

James Griffith
November 2022

Warming up
Introduction

Athletics. 2021. The Tokyo Olympics finally begin, but a year late as a result of the coronavirus pandemic. Team GB are energised and there are high hopes of medals after the successful World Championships in Doha in 2019. One of these defending champions, Katarina Johnson-Thompson, steps up to the starting line of the 200 metres – one of her strongest events of the heptathlon. She is leading at the bend, but then disaster strikes as she begins to slow down dramatically and starts limping. After being offered help, Johnson-Thompson refuses, climbs back up and practically hops to the finish line. It was heartbreak for Katarina Johnson-Thompson, but also a 'miracle' she crossed the finish line, as we discover she started the year in a wheelchair having ruptured her Achilles the previous December. By summer 2022, the Commonwealth Games gold medal will be placed round her neck.

Cricket. 2019. The England selectors and team captain Eoin Morgan have chosen their squad for the Cricket World Cup of 2019 to be held in England and Wales. They agonised over the choices of players to make up this squad, but equally important to their success was his choice of backroom staff: the analysts, coaches, doctor and physiotherapist.

Most people associate physiotherapy with sport and the injuries of high-profile sportsmen and women. For instance, it is not uncommon on a Monday morning, when flicking through the back pages of the paper, to see that Johnny X is being assessed by the physiotherapist after having sustained a knock in the weekend's Premiership match. It is a physiotherapist's job to rehabilitate the multi-million-pound stars from their bumps and cuts (and broken bones, torn ligaments, muscle damage, etc.).

At the other end of the scale, physiotherapy can be used to correct smaller injuries, for example those sustained in an accident when the victim needs to learn to walk properly again. It has also gained prominence as a profession because of the leading role it has taken in the armed forces and the rehabilitation work it does with soldiers who have been injured in the line of duty, allowing them to lead normal lives after what are life-altering injuries, and this work needs to be reflected.

In short, physios are invaluable.

Never before has physiotherapy been so much in the media attention; whether from initiatives to get the UK moving and deal with growing health issues, or with physiotherapists having an increased role in the management of a sports team with power of veto and sports stars being suspended for arguing with their decisions. There are also the difficulties the profession faces, with issues ranging from an ageing population to the rise in obesity, to cuts in services. There are many other facets to the profession outside of the treatment room, and admissions tutors require you to be fully aware of that.

I regularly counsel students on their A level subject choices in line with their talents and their desired onward university degree. Few are aware of how competitive physiotherapy is, particularly as they may be weighing this degree choice up against something else like medicine. I hope this book will provide a better understanding on the benefits of studying physiotherapy at undergraduate level and how to make a competitive application in order to obtain a place.

Physiotherapy is a popular degree, and some universities have cut the number of places on offer, meaning that there is now even greater competition for places. Table 1 (below) shows you approximately how many applicants there are per place for a few selected universities. There has been little change in this data over the past few years.

University	Applicants per place (approx.)
Birmingham	9
Bradford	22
Cardiff	17
East Anglia	16
East London	10
Hertfordshire	13
Huddersfield	12
King's College London	16
Kingston (delivered with St George's, University of London)	9
Liverpool	20
Robert Gordon	13
Sheffield Hallam	12
Southampton	36
Teesside	33
Ulster	12

Source: HEAP 2024 University Degree Course Offers (Trotman Education).
Table 1: Number of applicants per place at this selection of universities

What is physiotherapy?

The human body is a complex machine that can go wrong for any number of reasons. Physiotherapy is a science-based medical subject that looks in detail at how the body moves; how muscles, bones, joints and ligaments work and how they react to pain and trauma. Physiotherapists diagnose numerous ailments that affect the muscles and nerves, and then proceed to treat the patient, ensuring independence, movement and a return to maximum performance. It is the physiotherapist's job not only to look at the problem and treat it but also to look for any predisposing factors that may have contributed to the patient's ailment and to advise on how to minimise the risk of the same thing happening again.

Qualified physiotherapists work both independently and as part of multidisciplinary teams, ensuring that patients' health and mobility are improved.

What do physiotherapists do?

Physiotherapists have numerous challenging roles within the health sector. They provide services such as rehabilitation and exercise before and after surgery. Within the wider community they provide services to adults with learning difficulties. They also have a role in the workplace, where they can help to reduce injuries such as repetitive strain injury (RSI).

Chartered physiotherapists work with a wide range of people in many different environments, either individually or as part of a large healthcare team.

Physiotherapists deal with many different situations, including the following:

- patient education. This is very important in physiotherapy and means teaching people the 'correct' way to move and lift in order to prevent or slow the onset of problems such as back pain or RSI (see Chapter 7). This may include helping athletes to avoid injury by discussing techniques and training programmes. Poor warm-up routines, too much training, poor equipment and incorrect technique are common causes of injuries, and all of these can be avoided. Using the idea that prevention is better than cure, physiotherapists are able to show people that very small changes will be hugely beneficial: for example, good footwear, or the use of a wrist support when using a computer.
- helping women before and after pregnancy by advising them about posture and exercise

- helping children to deal with mental and physical disabilities
- developing the potential of people with learning difficulties through exercise, sport and recreation; this could also include the use of specialist equipment
- helping stroke victims to recover movement in paralysed limbs
- helping heart attack victims to reduce the risk of future recurrence
- helping orthopaedic patients after spinal operations or joint replacements and treating those debilitated following an accident. Using a variety of techniques to strengthen muscles and improve the mobility of individual joints, activities such as walking can be made much easier for people recovering from hip replacements or those with arthritis or osteoporosis. These methods can also reduce the pain and stiffness resulting from these conditions.
- working with AIDS patients
- caring for those people who suffer from Parkinson's disease (one in 37 people in the UK will be diagnosed with Parkinson's disease at some point in their life)
- helping people to deal with stress and anxiety
- improving the confidence and self-esteem of those with mental illness through exercise and recreation, while also helping with relaxation and body-awareness techniques
- working with the terminally ill (both inpatients and outpatients) or those in intensive care to maintain movement and prevent respiratory problems
- helping sportspeople recover from injury
- working in large businesses and companies to ensure that employees do not suffer from physical problems associated with their jobs.

Physiotherapists use a range of techniques, including:

- exercise
- hydrotherapy (see Glossary)
- infrared and ultraviolet radiation (see Glossary)
- manipulation
- massage
- ultrasound (see Glossary)
- vibration
- patient education
- movement analysis
- gait re-education (see Glossary)
- heat and cold application.

About this book

This book is structured very much like a standard physiotherapy session: it requires adequate warm-up, intensive drills and jumping through hoops, before finally seeing the finishing line, only for you to be given a leaflet detailing specific exercises for you to do at home. Stretch and challenge your mind, without breaking your back!

How to use this book

The competition for places on approved degree courses is intense – there are very few university courses other than physiotherapy that have more applicants per place. Typically, a university might receive over 1,000 applications for 40 places. Even if each applicant makes five choices – and not all do – this still works out at around five students chasing every place. As you have seen on page 2, the numbers are often far higher than this. With such intense competition for places you need to think carefully about all the stages of your application: from the preparation that you do before you apply, through to the interview. You should also think about the steps you can take to maximise your chances of gaining a place should something go wrong at the examination stage.

This book covers the following:

1. what physiotherapists do
2. getting an interview
3. getting an offer
4. results day
5. useful information.

The book begins with outlining what physiotherapists do, and looks at the kind of career you can expect as a physiotherapist. It also describes what the study of physiotherapy involves and the different course structures on offer. Please note that this book is designed to be a route map for potential physiotherapists rather than a comprehensive guide to physiotherapy as a profession. The Chartered Society of Physiotherapy, or physiotherapists you meet during work experience, should be the starting points for more detailed information on what being a physiotherapist entails.

The book then goes on to deal with the preparation that you need to undertake in order to make your application as strong as possible. It includes advice on work experience, how to choose a university and the UCAS application itself. Information for students with Scottish Highers, the International Baccalaureate (IB), the BTEC National Diploma or the Irish Leaving Certificate is on page 36.

It then covers interviews and provides tips on what to expect and on how to ensure that you come across as a potential physiotherapist. The book also contains a checklist for you to tick off the important steps in making your application.

The 'Results day' chapter describes the steps that you need to take if you are holding an offer, or if you do not have an offer but want to gain a place through Clearing. In Chapter 9 there is advice and information for 'non-standard' applicants – mature students, graduates and retake students.

Further to this, the book provides useful information on fees and funding and details of the universities offering courses, including their entry requirements. The universities will be happy to provide you with further information on other qualifications.

To conclude, there is a further information section and a glossary. Here you will find details of sources of further information on physiotherapy and definitions of any terms and abbreviations relevant to your UCAS application for physiotherapy courses.

1 | Pressure points
Careers

The book's aim is to make sure that you are completely well versed with the fundamentals of physiotherapy before you apply for university study; that includes knowing about the different career opportunities available to you in this profession. The field you are hoping to enter offers a great deal of options and exciting pathways.

It is equally important, when you have qualified for the profession, that you are quite open-minded in your approach and progressive in terms of your thinking. Physiotherapists normally work autonomously, as they are able to accept referrals from a range of sources (though professional autonomy is only granted to Chartered Society of Physiotherapy (CSP) members) and therefore you have to consider the business elements of the profession, i.e. balancing treatment with an understanding of how to balance the books. What this means is that physiotherapists make their own clinical judgements and treatment decisions and they also work in reflection, i.e. reviewing themselves and making corrections to their work where necessary.

Physiotherapy is a career that relies on the strength of the individual as well as the ability to work in a team. Physiotherapy as a subject is highly academic and therefore of great value; this means that employment prospects are large and varied. These prospects are not limited to the NHS; there is an enormous breadth of employment prospects that can be found across the different sectors (see pages 9–11).

Physiotherapy is not, however, a profession that involves only physical therapy. Physiotherapists work with people – in most cases people who are disabled, or who have been ill or injured. Physiotherapists need to be able to communicate on a personal level with people of all ages; to be reassuring and comforting; to explain the treatments they are using; and to help patients overcome fear and pain. Physiotherapists need to be able to assess the needs of their patients and to be aware of the effects of external circumstances such as social or cultural factors.

Working as a physiotherapist

Physiotherapists work in a wide range of health and care environments that include hospitals, the local community, private practice, industry and sports settings. The NHS is the largest employer of physiotherapists in the UK. Physiotherapy comprises the largest group within the allied healthcare professions, with approximately 63,000 state-registered physiotherapists in the UK, which compares to 42,000 just ten years ago.

A typical working day depends on whether you are working in the NHS or private practice. In the majority of cases, physiotherapists work in hospitals with normal working days, i.e. 9am–5pm, Monday–Friday. There are occasions when a weekend may be required, but this is symptomatic of the health professions.

The most identifiable example is of a hospital physiotherapist working in the Physiotherapy Department. A calendar booking system is in operation, as in a GP surgery, where they will see many patients per day, each one for an allotted period of time, about a range of problems, such as rehabilitation from broken bones, bad backs and arthritis, for a range of ages.

Those working in hospitals might work on the wards and visit the ward staff to discuss the treatment plans of new patients. Sometimes they then treat them as part of their ongoing care, often taking them to the physiotherapy department. A ward physiotherapist might have half a dozen wards to cover, varying from children's wards, to orthopaedic wards or stroke units. In some cases, a physiotherapist might be required to work in the intensive care unit if it is thought essential to the immediate rehabilitation of a patient.

Physiotherapists in private practice may have more opportunities to travel, depending on the job they are doing. If you work for a professional sporting association, for example, you may find that you have to travel a lot to support the team. Sometimes patients will be referred to you, other times you will need to target your business, and that may require advertising.

The concept of travel is also becoming more common in the NHS as a result of changes, as physiotherapists are doing more home visits to support the elderly.

To qualify as a registered physiotherapist you need to gain an approved degree (see page 17) that has been validated by the CSP and the Health & Care Professions Council (HCPC). If you complete the degree you must then register with the HCPC to use the professional title of physiotherapist and you are eligible for membership of the Chartered Society of Physiotherapy (CSP).

As with any career, there are pros and cons to physiotherapy. It is up to you to decide if the pros outweigh the cons. That is why work experience is invaluable, as it will either confirm your decision to pursue the career or demonstrate to you that you should seek an alternative occupation. Physiotherapists have a lot of demands on their time and they often can be stretched to the limit – if you will excuse the pun – because of the nature of their work, especially within the NHS, where, as a result of staffing cuts, there is more work for an individual physiotherapist. However, the variety and nature of the work is what physiotherapists thrive on and it is a hugely rewarding career, as you get to see the continuing progress of an individual patient over time.

The question of what attributes a physiotherapist needs is a common one. It is easy to say 'be physically fit'; at the end of the day, practise what you teach. Not to be flippant, it is a good point, as in any very demanding job that requires you to be on your feet most of the day, you want to make sure that you are looking after yourself. Additionally, you also need to consider the psychology of the patient. As with the relationship between a client and a personal trainer in a gym, a patient will have more confidence in their instructor if they can see that the instructor takes good care of themselves. Being active is also necessary for clear thinking, as it gives you the energy to get through the week.

However, over and above that, there are other characteristics that define a good physiotherapist. You need to have patience, peace of mind, the strength of character to encourage a patient and firmness to make sure that they achieve their targets. A physiotherapist is a strategist. Each individual one will find their own style – and you should be encouraged to find yours – but it all comes from this foundation and you need to consider now whether you possess those attributes.

Common career paths for physiotherapists

Once you have completed your BSc in Physiotherapy you will, hopefully, gain membership of the CSP and become registered with the HCPC – all degree courses in the UK are now accredited by the CSP and the HCPC. To say that there is a standard route is not correct. The main thing you need after graduating is clinical experience, and the usual route will be to gain experience in areas that you did not cover on your placements, usually as a junior in a rotational band 5 job with a starting salary of around £27,055.

A rotational band 5 job is a general physiotherapist role in which you rotate through the various departments in a hospital, including respiratory, stroke, orthopaedic, etc. Each rotation will last around four months. These are commonly in the NHS or in some private practices and are designed to build up your expertise before you can qualify for the next band (band 6). These bands also equate to your pay scale.

A lot of physiotherapists get their rotational band 5 job through the NHS or by having impressed on their placements during their course. However, you do not have to have worked for the NHS first before going into private practice. Some physiotherapists set up their own practices, but their success is all based on reputation and on building up the relevant experience over many years. As for anything in life, you have to prove yourself first.

Further qualifications are not essential after your degree, but you are expected to maintain your continuing professional development, which is very important and discussed below.

Private practice is one of the more lucrative career moves. Private practice, as an umbrella term, includes:

- treating patients independently for the same ailments as in the NHS
- working for a sports club or a specific team, aiding in the recovery of sportspersons from injury and helping to optimise their performance
- occupational rehabilitation, which means helping people to recover from accidents or illnesses and to return to their normal lives.

There are also additional opportunities to go off on a tangent and get involved in policy development and research, in order to ensure that physiotherapy as a profession continues to progress over time in line with NHS changes and guidelines.

Some of the other areas of work available to you as an aspiring physiotherapist are outlined in Table 2.

Area	Work
Animal physiotherapist	Supporting animals with the rehabilitation process following a medical operation.
Higher education lecturer	Lecturing on physiotherapy in universities or further education colleges.
Sports therapists	Rehabilitating and providing treatment on sporting injuries, educating athletes and giving advice on prevention.
Acupuncturist	Maintenance of patient health through the process of acupuncture.
Chiropractor	Treating patients through physical manipulation, massage, and rehabilitative exercise.

Table 2: Areas of work for physiotherapists

Area	Work
Dance movement psychotherapist	Using dance as a method to develop individuals mentally and emotionally.
Exercise physiologist	Providing scientific support to athletes and sports teams.
Health service manager	Operational responsibility within a hospital, GP surgery or community health service.
Health improvement practitioner	Encouraging lifestyle and behavioural changes to improve overall health and wellbeing.
Osteopath	Treatment of various musculoskeletal health issues.
Personal trainer	Helping others to achieve their fitness goals, more commonly within a gym setting.

Table 2: Continued

Employment prospects

In 2019, the CSP reported: 'There is a serious shortage of physiotherapists in England, caused by insufficient numbers of physiotherapy student places at a time of growing demand. This is creating difficulties in recruiting physiotherapists. A minimum of 500 additional physiotherapists need to be trained each year ... to meet the current shortfall.'

At that time, the Home Office had not included physiotherapy in the Shortage Occupation List. Fortunately, the CSP continued to lobby for this and physiotherapists were added to the shortage occupation list in 2021. This addition is key as it will enable businesses and public services to reach talent on a global scale. This should ultimately improve the employability prospects for both domestic and international students.

What is important to note is that significantly more physiotherapists are registered with the HCPC than are employed with the NHS. A growing proportion (approximately 32,000) of physiotherapists work outside the NHS (for example, in private hospitals, sports clubs or their own private practice), and these are more difficult to track, as the statistics rely on the voluntary registration to the HCPC of physiotherapists. In 2021, 60% of CSP members employed by the NHS considered or pursued non-NHS employment within the 12 months prior, while a further 20% actively sought to move out of the NHS. The number of vacancies within the NHS has consequently more than tripled between September 2019 and September 2021.

In the last CSP membership review (2021), there were 74% female to 26% male physiotherapists. Physiotherapists have a relatively young age profile, with 57% of CSP members being under 40 years of age; this is key as it shows a surge in retirement is not expected.

You can maximise your chances of employment by studying for a degree accredited by the CSP and HCPC and also by being a student member of the CSP.

> *'My main drive for wanting to become an accredited physiotherapist was the desire to help people and provide them with the knowledge of how to better look after their bodies after an injury. I've always been interested in physiology and how the body works and repairs itself after trauma. Being a keen runner who has represented both my school and university in the 800 metres and 1500 metres, I naturally researched my injuries and how I could best avoid repeating them! I always envisaged myself working with athletes or maybe for a professional sports club after completing my BSc in Physiotherapy, but now I'm not so sure. From my placements at the local hospital, through my course, I now have a much wider knowledge of what it means to be a physiotherapist and the varying fields you can work in. The pleasure I have got from working and helping people with long-term disabilities such as cerebral palsy or chronic physical conditions has shown me where my future career lies. I would therefore advise anyone who wants to become a physiotherapist to go into the profession with an open mind and see the discipline as a whole; rather than just focussing on one area that initially appeals to them. Who knows what you may end up doing?'*
>
> Monica, London South Bank University

To give you an indication of what pay you could be expecting if you joined the physiotherapy profession, starting salaries for qualified physiotherapists (Band 5) range from £27,055 to £32,934. Senior physiotherapists can earn between £33,706 and £40,588 (Band 6). As a clinical specialist/team leader, you can earn between £41,659 and £47,672 (Band 7). Salaries for advanced practice, extended scope or clinical lead physiotherapists range from £48,526 to £54,619 (Band 8a). Salaries rise to in excess of £67,064 (Band 8c) for management roles, such as head of service. For a more detailed breakdown of salaries and bands please visit: www.healthcareers.nhs.uk/working-health/working-nhs/nhs-pay-and-benefits/agenda-change-pay-rates.

As physiotherapists progress in their careers, they are expected to keep up to date with the Continuing Professional Development (CPD) framework detailed below. As they do this and achieve higher levels of responsibility – and indeed reach team leadership and management roles – they have the opportunity to increase their earnings.

The NHS has a structured tiering of pay grades and you will need to follow their framework in order to move up the scales. However, private practice is of course different, with remuneration determined by market forces, such as competition and demand. In-house private physiotherapy, such as in sports clubs for example, will determine the pay scales themselves. However, pay is always determined by experience and therefore the more emphasis you put on CPD, the quicker you will progress in your career.

Continuing Professional Development

Throughout their careers, physiotherapists are expected to develop their skills and to keep up to date with developments within the field in a structured and systematic way. This is known as continuing professional development (CPD). Physiotherapists are responsible for identifying, planning and recording their own CPD, setting themselves targets and collecting evidence in a portfolio to support their CPD. The process of CPD is summarised in Figure 1.

Occupational therapy

While there are a number of differences between physiotherapy and occupational therapy, a lot of similarities are also found. The link is often between dealing with the physical and the mental faculties of a patient in order to ensure their overall rehabilitation. Occupational therapists help people to carry out the tasks and activities that are necessary for them to lead a fulfilling life. These might be work related – helping people with disabilities to cope with their jobs – or they might be everyday things such as cooking, bathing, travelling or socialising. Occupational therapists work in hospitals, for charities and social organisations, in schools and the workplace, in prisons, within the local community and in many other situations. Occupational therapists deal with physical, mental and social needs, for example:

- helping children deal with learning difficulties
- helping people with mental illness to look after themselves, or to be successful in their jobs
- working with accident victims to enable them to re-learn physical tasks
- advising businesses about how to adapt facilities and premises to enable people with disabilities to cope with their jobs
- creating rehabilitation programmes for refugees or the homeless.

To practise as an occupational therapist, it is necessary to follow a degree course, either undergraduate or postgraduate, in occupational therapy which has been approved by the Health & Care Professions Council (HCPC) and accredited by the Royal College of Occupational Therapists (RCOT). Graduates seeking international experience may seek a degree which is also approved by the World Federation of Occupational Therapy (WFOT).

Contact details for the RCOT and other useful organisations can be found on pages 103–104.

```
┌─────────────────────────────────────┐
│   Identify areas for improvement    │
└─────────────────────────────────────┘
                  ↓
┌─────────────────────────────────────┐
│   Collect evidence for portfolio    │
└─────────────────────────────────────┘
                  ↓
┌─────────────────────────────────────┐
│          Evaluate outcomes          │
└─────────────────────────────────────┘
                  ↓
┌─────────────────────────────────────┐
│   Activities to achieve these goals │
└─────────────────────────────────────┘
                  ↓
┌─────────────────────────────────────┐
│           Identify goals            │
└─────────────────────────────────────┘
                  ↓
┌─────────────────────────────────────┐
│           Related courses           │
└─────────────────────────────────────┘
```

Figure 1: Process of continuing professional development (CPD)

Case study: Harvey, first-year student at University of East Anglia

Harvey's parents were doctors but his father always wanted him to find his own career path. Harvey had looked into medicine, but decided that it was not the right career for him, based on work experience that he had had. However, a chance placement through a family contact led to him work-shadowing a physiotherapist as part of his school's work experience week.

'That opportunity was revolutionary for me in terms of my future. I had always wanted to do something from a basis of care but medicine and dentistry just did not appeal and I have too many allergies to animals for veterinary science. However, joking aside, I remember one particular patient who inspired me the most. This man had overcome so much adversity after an accident whereby he had broken both of his legs and had been in traction for a year, as well as disturbing his spine to the extent that it was believed he would not walk again. I saw how the physio dealt with him and through his own sheer strength of will, he was slowly turning around that prognosis and forcing himself to learn how to walk again. The role of the physio just cannot be understated in that example.

'So I set about focusing my A levels on my future goal. Though that was not easy, as there are no definite subjects you should choose, apart from a biological science. Therefore, I focused on the subjects I was good at because ultimately you need strong grades. I took ancient history, biology, chemistry and drama and theatre studies, the latter of which should not be scoffed at because it has built my confidence and interaction levels.

'When I was applying for universities, I looked at the entrance requirements of many universities and also rang many of them to get a clear steer on work experience. Following their advice, I spent my A level year and summer holiday taking on a variety of placements to give me a complete picture of the profession and to start building my skills. I firmly believe this is what got me my interviews, as the majority of questions they asked me centred on the work. They quizzed me on what I had learnt and gave me a couple of scenarios to see what my instinctive response would be. I enjoyed the interviews but they were looking to see whether what I had said I had actually completed.

'I learnt so much before I even started my course, from the glamour of certain physiotherapy, to the emotionally resilient work in stroke units. I am very much looking forward to graduating but there is a lot of hard work ahead. My best advice to anyone thinking of physiotherapy is that you can never be too prepared, as the competition is tough. Also, research the universities and their courses. They are all different and will be suited to some but not everyone. Find where you think the course will most benefit you.'

Harvey went to the University of East Anglia after achieving AAA in his A levels.

2 | Strengthen your core
Physiotherapy courses: what to expect

This chapter deals with the types of course that you can expect at university. It looks at the typical structure of a BSc as well as the different teaching approaches you might find. It also discusses courses in Scotland, Wales and Northern Ireland and the differences in course style, as well as MSc (pre-registration) courses. It is useful to note that these are guidelines and that courses can vary between universities, so make sure you research the available courses properly.

In the UK, as mentioned in the previous chapter, a physiotherapist requires a degree from a CSP/HCPC-accredited course in order to practise with confidence. In turn, if you practise in the UK, you are required by law to be registered with the HCPC. An accredited three-year degree will allow you to register with the HCPC and CSP after graduation. All undergraduate physiotherapy degree programmes in the UK at mainstream universities are accredited by the CSP.

Physiotherapy is a very competitive course and, as such, the entry levels will be set higher than the minimum. For many universities, there are no prescribed A levels that you should take, unlike for medicine, although some universities do request biology (or human biology). Others might request one or two scientific subjects more broadly, so you should still carefully consider what to study for your A Levels, e.g. psychology would be better as a third subject than film studies. Physical education or sports science is often listed as a requirement, either as an alternative to or in addition to biology. Top GCSE grades (7–9/A–B) are highly desirable, and you will need to achieve competitive A level results, usually in the A–B grade bracket, depending on the academic establishment, with AAA–ABB being a typical offer. However, always bear in mind that entry requirements from universities are the minimum. A lot of people will be applying with higher predicted grades and there is also much more to the application than academic achievement, which we will discuss later in the book.

The key for now is to check each individual university's website in order to find out the details you require.

Typical course structure

In accordance with good practice set out by the HCPC, all UK physiotherapy courses are revalidated every five to seven years. While all physiotherapy courses contain many common elements, there are significant differences in the structure of courses, in the course content, in the way in which the practical and patient-contact elements are arranged and in the styles of assessment. You should investigate this thoroughly by reading prospectuses and looking at the physiotherapy departments' websites in order to find out which ones will suit you best.

In a continuing move towards the development of physiotherapy in the community and the focus on prevention, many universities have adjusted their course to reflect this and to help students meet the changing state of the NHS and be able to work successfully within it.

Example course structure: Brunel University London

Year 1

- Anatomy 1: Lower Quadrant
- Anatomy 2: Upper Quadrant
- Continuing Professional Development 1
- Musculoskeletal Lower Quadrant 1
- Pathophysiology
- Rehabilitation 1 and 2
- Respiratory

Year 2

- Cardiovascular Health
- Clinical Preparation 1
- Continuing Professional Development 2
- Musculoskeletal 2: Upper Quadrant
- Neurorehabilitation
- Physiotherapy Practice 1: Ageing Studies
- Physiotherapy Practice 2: Paediatrics
- Placements 1 and 2
- Research Methods

Year 3

- Continuing Professional Development 3
- Critical Care
- Physiotherapy Practice 3: Women's Health
- Physiotherapy Practice 4: Oncology & Palliative Care
- Physiotherapy Practice 5: Emerging Practice

2   Physiotherapy courses: what to expect

- Physiotherapy Practice 6: Mental Health
- Placements 3, 4 and 5
- Professional Practice
- Research Proposal

*Source: www.brunel.ac.uk/study/undergraduate/physiotherapy-bsc.
Reprinted with kind permission of Brunel University London.*

Research dissertation

There will be continuing modules in research alongside the clinical placements. Evidence-based practice is essential in physiotherapy, therefore students need to learn how to carry out research as well as how to use existing research. For all honours degrees, this is a major component of the course in the second and third years, and there is a focus towards a research dissertation that will be submitted in the final year. This part of the course enables you to manage and organise a research project. You will choose an area of interest in the field of physiotherapy. Here you will consolidate and develop your analytical skills and critically evaluate found evidence. Most dissertations will be around 10,000 words in length.

Elective clinical placement

At the end of the third year there may be an elective clinical placement. You will choose the specialty in which you wish to work and arrange the placement yourself. Many students choose to work abroad, or in areas of healthcare not previously encountered in their own clinical education.

Be aware of the different teaching styles of the courses and refer to the universities' websites to find all the information. Some courses are modular, some have a lot of emphasis on clinical teaching and others are more theoretical. You need to find out which courses best suit your needs, offer you the opportunities you seek and that will help you flourish.

Teaching styles

These will be different, depending on the instructor and the course material; however, they can broadly be split into the following types.

- **Interactive:** An interactive style is what the name implies, with discussions, Q&A sessions and presentations. This style suits those who have already absorbed the facts, and students will

pursue independent research and build on this through the practical aspects of the course.
- **Lecture:** A lecture is useful for providing a lot of facts in one session, which will then be researched further outside the course. This implies extra reading to supplement what you have been taught.
- **Problem-based learning (PBL):** This is student-centred learning where you will learn about topics by looking at multifaceted and realistic problems. You will work in groups and identify what you know, what you need to know and how you will find the information necessary for solving the problems. The instructor will ask questions and provide resources to lead you to the right answers. However, you must figure the answers out for yourself.
- **Practice-based professional learning (PBPL):** This style requires a level of professional practice in order to fully understand the course. It is in contrast to theory-led learning and is directly related to the practical aspects of the course. It is a new style of learning and is prevalent in the newer universities.

You should look on the websites for the individual universities to find out which teaching styles they use. See Chapter 11 for university contact details.

Courses in Scotland

There are three universities in Scotland where you can study physiotherapy.

1. Queen Margaret University, Edinburgh.
2. Glasgow Caledonian University.
3. Robert Gordon University, Aberdeen.

The courses are four years full time, rather than three years full time as in England. The courses have a strong clinical bias, with work placements, and you are required to complete an honours project in your fourth year.

It is also possible to take a two-year MSc in Physiotherapy pre-registration course after taking a different degree. This allows students another opportunity to study physiotherapy after having studied in a different but scientifically related discipline.

The section below summarises the options on offer on the Scottish courses so that you can see the different approaches of a Scottish university. Apart from the length of course, you will see that they are not wholly dissimilar to the English courses.

Queen Margaret University

Year 1 is spent learning the basic and applied sciences needed for physiotherapy. Year two begins to focus more on cardiorespiratory, musculoskeletal and neurological physiotherapy. In the final year, you will complete a research project with the support of a project supervisor.

Part of your learning will be alongside an experienced, registered physiotherapist, working with patients, carers and/or families. It is important to work with other health and social care professionals to see the role each plays in a patient's care. Practice-based learning is employed in settings around Scotland; this is funded by you. It may be possible to take one optional practice-based placement overseas.

Glasgow Caledonian University

The aim of this course is to give you the professional and academic knowledge and skills needed to manage individual patients. This course promotes your critical analysis skills, which you will have to use to justify and evaluate evidence in your practical work. This will be particularly relevant in your honours project in the fourth year. You will also visit clinical simulation labs, take field trips, have educational placements and use e-learning. There is scope to gain experience in a placement in the UK or abroad. Students will undertake at least 1,000 hours of supervised practice placement experience during their study. Healthy lifestyles and physical activity are promoted heavily on this course and placements play a big part in supplementing your learning.

Robert Gordon University

A very modern course, this is designed to help you 'meet the demands of the rapidly changing health sector'. The clinical placement is of primary importance, as it gives you the 'real' experiences that will ensure your professional credibility.

This is very much a practical course, with a high proportion of practical assessment within the first two years. The faculty building offers state-of-the-art teaching and clinical skills facilities. You will use practical therapy rooms and a human performance laboratory. There is also a 'sophisticated three-dimensional motion analysis system' that will allow you to see in action what it is you are being taught. There is also a unique, computerised 'METIMan' in the clinical skills area where you will be able to practise before going into a real-life setting.

The final year will put most emphasis on evaluation and research skills and two final clinical placements to refine the necessary techniques required for the profession.

Courses in Wales

The section below summarises the three-year, full-time options on offer at Cardiff University and Glyndŵr University. If you study physiotherapy at either of these universities and agree to work in Wales for two years upon completion of your studies, you may be eligible to receive the NHS Wales Bursary – this means that your tuition fees are paid and you will receive an annual £1,000 grant payment.

Alternatively, the University of South Wales offers a part-time physiotherapy degree of 4 years or longer.

Cardiff University

The department is over 100 years old and offers a CSP-accredited degree over three years. The diversity and complexity of the profession are mirrored in the theory and practice elements on this course. It combines university lectures with seven four-week placements spread across years 2 and 3. You will learn from both academic and clinical physiotherapists, creating a holistic approach. Students gain experience in all of the core areas of the profession. Placements take place around Wales but may also be arranged in other locations in order to maintain high standards. The university endeavours to provide students with extra-curricular opportunities, most notably volunteering their skills to support the annual Cardiff Half Marathon.

Glyndŵr University, Wrexham

Studies during the first year lay down the foundation knowledge and skills of problem-solving and clinical reasoning. A four-week placement provides an opportunity for students to reflect on the learning and prepare for Level 5 placement experience. Year 2 develops knowledge and skills in greater depth through studies in cardiorespiratory, neurology and the spine, and provides a six-week placement to consolidate the skills and knowledge from years 1 and 2. Year 3 offers increased opportunities for independent learning and self-reflection in preparation for employment.

2 Physiotherapy courses: what to expect

Courses in Northern Ireland

The section below summarises the options on offer at the University of Ulster.

University of Ulster

In Northern Ireland there is one principal university recognised by the CSP teaching the physiotherapy course, the University of Ulster. As in the other universities discussed above, there is a split between theory and practice, but a large emphasis is placed on practice-based learning. Applicants will also be video interviewed as part of the admissions process.

In years 1 and 2 of the programme, you will usually take at least six modules, including inter-professional modules. In the final year, students will undertake either an investigative project or a dissertation. A feature of this course is the integration of theory and practice; participation is expected from everyone and peer examination is used as a testing device. The University of Ulster uses practice-based learning. Beginning in your first year, you will take part in five clinical placements during the course, totalling 30 weeks, to help confirm your learning.

MSc (pre-registration) course

This is different from the postgraduate MSc in Physiotherapy, which is for students who have already trained as a physiotherapist and now want to specialise. The MSc (pre-registration) course, for students who have not yet trained in physiotherapy, is a two-year, full-time qualifying programme for graduates with a suitable and relevant first degree. This would usually be a scientific subject based around biology, i.e. biology, behavioural science, physiology, etc. (This course is arguably even more competitive than the BSc entry, because of both the number of applicants and the demands placed on you.) The course fees are £9,250 in English universities (slightly higher in Scottish universities), and there is a means-tested NHS-funded bursary to help with living expenses. Fees for EU/international students are much more variable, and it is therefore advisable that overseas applicants check the university webpages for fee information.

The course aims to give students with the necessary skills a second opportunity to take on evidence-based physiotherapy programmes with a variety of patients. A large emphasis is placed on the implementation of research and auditing programmes. This course is accredited by the CSP and the HCPC.

Course overview

The course is divided between research and clinical placements. A large emphasis is placed on the latter, which is typically arranged over six modules with over 1,000 hours of study. Students will treat patients and watch professionals in different settings, from in-house to home visits. There are three core areas: the management of neurological, cardiopulmonary and neuromusculoskeletal dysfunctions, with knowledge from the biomedical and psycho-social sciences recruited as required.

First year

The first year develops practice and reasoning in the core areas of practice. Evaluation and critical analysis are key to development in terms of physiotherapeutic concepts. In the last part of the year students begin their research project.

Second year

The clinical modules and research project continue during the second year. There will also be work on an Advancing Physiotherapy module, which addresses other approaches to the management of physiotherapy.

Practice placements

These are a key factor in the education of a physiotherapist, and will take place over the two-year study, usually occupying 1,000 hours in total. You will normally be seconded to a range of diverse and exciting placements, where you will gain a variety of experience with numerous client groups, under the guidance of skilled clinicians. Each student will gain experience of physiotherapy within various placement settings.

3 | Pulled in every direction
Work experience

According to the CSP:

> *'Gaining work experience is helpful but can be difficult to organise in physiotherapy because of current training pressures on relevant departments. However, work experience in any aspect of healthcare will be useful to you. This is because admissions tutors are looking for evidence that you can communicate well with all ages and sections of the community. Have a look into work experience and try: your local hospital and their physiotherapy department(s) (private or public); private physiotherapy clinics; sports clinics, football clubs, special schools and units (for disabled children and adults), and nursing homes; voluntary work (eg Red Cross Association, St Johns Ambulance Society, MS Society).'*
>
> Information taken from the CSP (www.csp.org.uk),
with kind permission from the CSP.

Work experience was previously vital in order to be considered for a place on many physiotherapy courses. However, since the coronavirus pandemic, at the time of writing universities are not expecting students to have been able to obtain work experience since March 2020, and have temporarily softened their stance on the need for work experience. If you do have such an opportunity though, preferably within the NHS, it will certainly put you at an advantage. It is your introduction to the profession at first hand, and evidence that you have worked with people in the community. For example, Brunel University's website (www.brunel.ac.uk) says that all applicants are advised to undertake an observational clinical experience' with a chartered physiotherapist; and St George's stresses that even though work experience requirements have been relaxed, they still require students 'to have an understanding of the realities of working as a healthcare professional and show they have the necessary skills and attributes for their chosen career.' They go on to advise online resources as an alternative way to seek this insight.

If you are very lucky (and very determined) you may be able to get a paid job in an NHS hospital as a physiotherapy assistant. However, because of school or college commitments, this is usually only possible during a gap year. It is more likely that you will have to settle for an unpaid volunteer position either on a part-time basis (at weekends or in the evenings) or for a short period of time in the school holidays.

Even before the pandemic, training pressures on hospital-based physiotherapy departments were making it difficult to get any relevant work experience; these pressure are even greater now, so anything within a health-related or care field will be very useful.

If you are unable to arrange any of the above, you should try to shadow a physiotherapist for a day or two, and supplement this with a volunteer job in another caring environment such as a hospice or special school. There are also a growing number of medicine-related summer schools and experiences that provide demonstrable insight into the profession.

Be fastidious in your investigation of how much work experience is required per institution. Some of the relaxations mentioned above may only be true at the time of writing, and as we move out of the pandemic, universities could quickly return to treating work experience as an essential requirement in order to obtain an offer. The universities' own websites are your starting place, followed by contacting the university directly if it does not publish the information.

Length of time

While there are no rules about the minimum length of time that you should spend doing work experience, volunteer work or work-shadowing, as a general rule those candidates who can demonstrate commitment by doing something on a regular basis throughout the year or who have spent at least two weeks in a hospital environment are likely to be in the strongest position. The current economic climate and the obstacles raised by the pandemic may require you to think outside the box. For example, you could volunteer in a care home or on a children's ward in a hospital and watch the nurses and physiotherapists there. You can also chat to physiotherapists or go to physiotherapy appointments with friends or relatives.

> 'Get as much experience as you can – it doesn't just have to be as a physiotherapy assistant. Be determined: there is always a way to get in if you really want to.'
>
> Katherine, University of Hertfordshire

Hospitals will often provide an opportunity for students to do a one-day work experience, and you should contact them directly regarding these opportunities.

Some schools operate schemes where they arrange work experience for you. This saves you the hard work of contacting hospitals or clinics, but the drawback is that you will be unable to impress the selectors with your dynamism and determination because you will not be able to say 'I arranged my work experience myself'.

How to apply

If your school does not operate such a scheme you have two options: to use any contacts that your family or friends have, or to approach local hospitals. To do the latter you need to get the names and addresses of local hospitals with physiotherapy departments and physiotherapy clinics from the internet. You should send an email to the hospital or clinic and include the name of a referee – someone who can vouch for your interest in physiotherapy as well as for your reliability. Your careers teacher, housemaster or housemistress or form teacher would be ideal. An example of a suitable email is given below.

> From: Rachel Thompson
> To: oakparkcare@wakeford.gov.uk
> Subject: Volunteering
>
> Dear Sir/Madam
>
> I am a Year 12 A level student interested in pursuing a career in physiotherapy. I plan to apply to study physiotherapy at university and am looking to gain as much experience as possible in this field. My interest in physiotherapy was sparked after attending an appointment with my grandmother after she sustained an injury. I was fascinated by the process of her recovery and though I have always enjoyed studying the sciences, I had never been inspired by a specific career before. I have heard that you are looking for volunteers and I would be delighted if you would consider me for a role. I am available at evenings and weekends so please let me know if you think this would be suitable for you. I am more than happy to discuss this further in person, and if you require a reference please contact my form tutor:
> Mr Shaw
> Featherstone Academy
> Wakeford
> WF8 7BY
> a.shaw@featherstone.ac.uk
>
> Thank you for your consideration.
>
> Yours sincerely,
> Rachel Thompson

When applying for work experience you will need to create a CV for the potential employers to get an idea of your skills and education. This is basically a summary of what you have done so far in your life to date. Within the CV will be your up-to-date contact details, educational qualifications and, of course, any previous work experience. Please see the sample CV below.

CV

Personal Details

Richard Hall
16 St Mary's Avenue
Peterborough
PE21 5TU
01733 523559
r.a.hall@zmail.co.uk

Education & Qualifications

2021–present: Kingswood High School, Peterborough
A levels: Biology, Chemistry, Physical Education
GCSEs (June 2021): Mathematics 8, English Language 8, English Literature 9, History 7, Physics 8, Chemistry 8, Biology 9, Spanish 7.

Work Experience

July 2022–present: High Street Book Shop, Peterborough.
Responsible for till work, replenishing stock from the storeroom, stocktaking and general duties.
October 2021–June 2022: Sales Assistant at local superstore. Duties included helping customers with their questions and needs. Also stocking shelves and some cashier work.

Skills

Languages – good written and spoken Spanish
Computing – competent in Word and Excel

Interests

I'm a keen cricket player and represent my local first team. I'm also interested in world cinema and a member of the school film club.

References

Mr J. Featherstone
Head of Sixth Form
Kingswood High School
Peterborough
j.featherstone@kingswood.ac.uk

Mrs K. Blake
Eastman's Bookshop
High Street
Peterborough
k.l.blake@eastmans.co.uk

As well as helping you to decide whether you are serious about physiotherapy and adding weight to your application, work experience is useful because you may be able to get one of the people you work with to give you a reference, which you could send in support of your UCAS application or produce at your interview.

Work experience in Wales

While you are at school or college, NHS Wales Informatics Service will support and help you decide on your next career move by offering work experience placements for one to 10 weeks. However, work placements can be hard to come by. It is very difficult, if not impossible, to get work experience in NHS Wales if you are under 18. The NHS Wales website that could be most helpful would be: www.wales.nhs.uk/ourservices/contactus/workvolunteeringandworkexperiencequestions.

Cardiff University and Glyndŵr University therefore do not stipulate work experience as being essential, but do want to see that applicants have spoken to physiotherapists or physiotherapy students, that they have looked at physiotherapy-related publications and they have contacted the CSP (which has a pretty comprehensive careers page). Cardiff University will interview all candidates, either by multiple mini interview (MMI) format, or online.

Things to look out for during work experience

The variety of treatments available to patients

Make sure that you know what you are observing. Ask the physiotherapist or nurse for the technical names of the procedures that you see, and for information on the techniques and equipment used. Ask about the advantages and disadvantages of different types of treatments, and in what situations they are used. Keep a diary of what you saw on a day-to-day basis so that you can use it to revise from prior to an interview. There are a number of websites that provide detailed information on medical conditions and treatments, and you could add further detail to your diary using one of these. See the list of 'Useful websites' at the end of the book (page 105).

Working as a physiotherapist

Ask the physiotherapist about his or her work life. Find out about the hours, the pay, the demands of the job and the career options open to physiotherapists. Find out what the physiotherapists like about the job and what they dislike.

> **Case study: Jessie, second-year student at University of Liverpool**
>
> 'Studying at Liverpool University for physiotherapy has been an amazing experience so far and one of my proudest achievements. Although coming straight from sixth form made me apprehensive initially, with perhaps less clinical experience than more mature students, I soon realised this wasn't a disadvantage. As a small cohort you get to know other students well and share experiences, while the lecturers encourage you and support you in the whole university experience.
>
> 'Many of our tutors are currently still employed in private or public practices, and they have provided opportunities and ideas for us outside of university lectures. Some of us have volunteered with local charities and hospitals, while external talks have provided an insight into different areas you can specialise in as a physiotherapist.
>
> 'We had about eight weeks out on practice in our first year of the course, with one week of this being an observational placement, which provided us the opportunity to put into perspective our knowledge at an early stage. All the other placements are six weeks at a time, divided evenly over the next few years to get over 1,000 hours on placement and become qualified. The university tries to get you a wide range of placements, such as respiratory, neurological, community and out-patient placements soon after covering those modules at university.
>
> 'Now in Year 2 of my physiotherapy course the intensity of study and research has increased. An average day starts at 10am and finishes at 5pm, with lunch and breaks. The day is usually split into two hours of theory in the morning, then putting this into "hands-on" practice in the afternoon, using each other as models, so you soon become comfortable with each other. There is always more work to do outside lecture hours, but this is manageable and there is time allocated for this.

'The physiotherapy lectures are mostly based on the campus. We have breaks between lectures and it's a good idea to consolidate our learning at the library; it has all of the resources you can wish for, and is a great place to study. Each project or assessment is different on the course, and so caters for all types of learners and enables a large range of skills for when we go out on placement.

'I'd say my most enjoyable side of physiotherapy so far is the time I spend with patients, as each assessment is different and to hear their stories of their accidents or condition is fascinating. I'm looking forward to studying outpatients and seeing how different this will be from what we have done before. After my completion of the course I have the next goal of securing a rotational band 5 physiotherapy position, which will lead on to securing a speciality area where I can begin my career and become the best physio I can be!'

Tips for work experience

- Dress as the physiotherapists dress: be clean, tidy and reasonably formal. There are no strict rules here. You should dress professionally – some wear a shirt and tie, in sports physiotherapy you might wear shorts and a polo shirt, and hospitals have their own specific uniforms. Use your common sense!
- Research the company that you are being interviewed by. What are their products? What is their history?
- Expand on your key skills and attributes.
- What times and dates are you available to work for them.
- Offer to help the physiotherapist or the nurses with routine tasks.
- Show an interest in everything that is going on around you.

'While my grandmother was in a care home in Leicestershire I enquired with the NHS management at the home if there was an opportunity for me to volunteer and help with the patients' physiotherapy. I was delighted that they agreed and I was able to help for about four hours per week. This experience showed me that I did indeed want to forge a career in physiotherapy. It also gave me great satisfaction: I was doing a job (even though voluntary) that had a massive positive effect on the people I was helping, and I gained so much valuable experience from the qualified team of physiotherapists who worked there.'

Ellen, University of Manchester

Discussing your work experience at interview

If you are fortunate enough to be called for interview then you can expect to discuss your work experience. It is a great way of an interviewer getting to know you and finding out more about your research. It would be a good idea to ask the employers where you volunteered to write a reference for you.

So, remember these golden points about the purpose of work experience to mention in the interview:

- confirmed your choice of study
- important for learning skills, which include: teamwork, independence, administration, etc.
- working hours
- care-based profession.

All the time with work experience, keep remembering what you are learning from the experience. The weakest applications are the ones that just mention work experience for the sake of it. There is nothing worse than a personal statement or interview with just a catalogue of work experiences but no substance behind them, as that is pure vanity. Work experience will form the basis of your discussions. Make some notes about what you learn as you go and take those notes with you on the day of your interview.

4 | On the rack/ under observation
The UCAS application

In order to gain a place at university you have to submit a UCAS application. Before you do this, however, you need to be sure that you have investigated physiotherapy as thoroughly as you can. You need to do this for two reasons.

1. You must be sure that physiotherapy is the right career for you.
2. You must demonstrate to the university admissions tutors that you are aware of the demands of the profession.

With so many applicants for every university place, the selectors need to be sure that they do not 'waste' a place on someone who will then drop out of the course or the profession. The number of applicants per place (approximate) varies, depending on the institution; for example, Birmingham has nine applicants for every place, whereas Southampton, at the opposite end of the scale, has 36 applicants for every place (see Table 1 on page 2). For this reason your application has to be very convincing. Most people's exposure to physiotherapy is limited, and so you need to investigate the profession in depth.

Choice of university

Once you have completed your work experience and are sure that you want to be a physiotherapist, you need to research your choice of university. There are various factors that you should take into account:

- the type of course
- the entrance requirements (see page 35)
- location
- whether you will be taught alongside students on other healthcare courses such as radiology, nursing, occupational therapy or podiatry.

Research

The first thing to do is to get hold of the prospectuses. If your school does not have spare copies, telephone the universities; they will send you a prospectus free of charge. You can also order these online, which is the quickest way of doing this, and most have a downloadable PDF for you to look at too. All universities have very informative websites that carry extra information on admissions policies.

> **TIP!**
>
> Do not simply select your universities because someone tells you that they have good reputations or that they are easier to get into, because you will be spending the next three or four years of your life at one of them, and if you do not like the place you are unlikely to last the course.

Apart from talking to current or former physiotherapy students or careers advisers, there are a number of other sources of information. The *Guardian* newspaper publishes its own league table of universities (www.theguardian.com/education/universityguide), ranked by a total score that combines the university's teaching assessment, a 'value added' score based on the class of degree obtained compared with A level (or equivalent) grades, spending on facilities and materials, student/staff ratios, job prospects and entrance requirements. *The Times* also compiles its own table, but this can only be accessed through a subscription payment. The Complete University Guide league table can be found at www.completeuniversityguide.co.uk/league-tables/rankings.

Other websites that are worth checking are the National Student Survey (www.thestudentsurvey.com), which gives existing undergraduate students a platform to share their experiences of colleges, courses and teaching. Also Discover Uni (discoveruni.gov.uk), which *'includes official statistics about higher education courses taken from national surveys and data collected from universities and colleges about their students'*.

Of course, league tables tell you only a small part of the whole story, and anyone who makes their choices solely on this basis without visiting the universities or reading the prospectuses is taking a serious risk.

Open days

Once you have narrowed down the number of universities to, say, seven or eight, you should try to visit them in order to get a better idea of what studying there would be like. Your school careers department will have details of open days (or you could telephone the universities directly). Equally, you can look on the websites and, for those that have the facility, use their online booking system for open days. Open days always get fully booked, so the earlier you do it, the better. Some universities will arrange for you to be shown around at other times of the year as well.

Going to open days also gives you the opportunity to ask an admissions tutor any questions that you might have about the university generally, such as about sporting activities, societies or accommodation. You should go with a list of questions and show yourself to be proactive. After all, you would not go shopping for clothes without trying them on! Details can be found on the university websites.

Several universities began to run online open days during the pandemic and most still offer virtual solutions in some capacity, such as virtual campus tours, live webinars and on-demand information videos. Many universities also now offer alumni chat functions on their websites, which can provide you with a different perspective on university life. While online events are more effective when it comes to the time and cost of travelling, it can be more difficult to gauge the feel of a campus and it's not so easy to ask questions.

Try to go to as many open days as you can, providing you are allowed to by your school. If you cannot attend the open day, go and have a look on another day and email any questions you have to the admissions tutor. Do not ask questions to which you can find answers for yourself on the website, such as 'What is the grade requirement?'; this does not show you to be proactive, just lazy. Ask for details, not generics.

Entrance requirements

Entrance requirements vary from university to university, but a 'standard' offer might ask for a minimum of ABB, with Russell Group universities often asking for AAB. The offer will probably specify that biology must be studied at A level, along with one other science. A* grades are not usually asked for but do represent higher points. It is most common that you will be given an offer based on getting three grades, as opposed to points. It is worthwhile checking your offer conditions when they come through, to see whether points are also accepted; offers expressed as points are usually minimum of 128 points from three A levels, or equivalent.

You should also check the university prospectuses for details of A level requirements. Some universities, for example, may specify that they require one of the subjects to be an arts subject or humanity, rather than them all being science subjects or mathematics.

If we take the University of Brighton's entry requirements as an example, then you will need to obtain ABB (128 UCAS points), including Biology, Human Biology or PE.

Other common qualifications that can also gain you access to courses are listed below:

Access to HE Diploma

A QAA-recognised Access to Science course which must include biological science. Pass with a minimum of 60 credits, 45 of which must be at level 3 (at least 30 distinctions and 15 merits).

BTEC Extended Diploma

DDM, and an A-level in Biology or Human Biology at grade B.

BTEC Higher National Diploma

DD in the BTEC National Diploma, to normally be accompanied by an A grade in a science A level.

Cambridge Pre-U

Combinations of three subjects allowed, normally including biology or PE, usually looking towards a D3/M1 or higher.

International Baccalaureate

34 points, with biology at Higher level.

Irish Leaving Certificate

Typically three As (A1–A2), three Bs (B1–B2) at Higher level, which must include Biology and English.

Scottish qualifications

Typically three As and two Bs at higher level, which must include Biology and English.

T levels

Merit in the Health T level; other T levels are not accepted.

The UCAS Tariff

The UCAS Tariff is the system for allocating points to qualifications used for entry to higher education.

The part that affects A level students is shown in Table 3 opposite.

However, what UCAS does say is that a lot of universities do not use the Tariff system and rely solely on grade offers; so do not worry unnecessarily about this Tariff, instead focus on getting those grades.*

*We acknowledge UCAS's contribution of this information.

4 The UCAS application

Qualification and Grade	UCAS Tariff
A level grade A*	56
A level grade A	48
A level grade B	40
A level grade C	32
A level grade D	24
A level grade E	16

Table 3: UCAS Tariff conversion chart

Your choices

There are five spaces in the UCAS application, all of which may be used for physiotherapy courses. (In contrast, students applying for medicine, dentistry or veterinary science may use only four of their five choices for such courses.) You do not have to fill all five spaces with physiotherapy courses. The key point to note here is that universities cannot see who else you have applied to and the order on the form is alphabetical, so you do not have to know your order from the outset. Only once you have got your offers will you put down Conditional Firm and Conditional Insurance. Therefore, you are allowed to apply for a mixture of physiotherapy courses and non-physiotherapy courses, or to leave spaces blank. Thus the important part is the personal statement as it must be written to reflect the course you are applying for at university. As all the courses have to be reflected in the same personal statement, they all have to be broadly similar in order to be sure that the personal statement can be tailored to each of your five choices without any ambiguity in terms of what you are applying for.

If you are worried that you might not be offered a place to study physiotherapy and you would consider other courses, you might want to put down four physiotherapy courses and one other course. The one non-physiotherapy course should be related to physiotherapy, either directly (occupational therapy, podiatry) or in a related discipline such as human biology, physiology. Other courses, such as radiology or nursing, are not related for example. You should not enter fewer than four physiotherapy courses in the application – if you do you are unlikely to convince the selectors that you are genuinely committed, not because they will know what other courses you have applied for, but because your personal statement will not reflect physiotherapy as much as it should.

> **TIP!**
>
> Applying for other courses such as medicine or veterinary science alongside your physiotherapy course should be avoided. It will be clear to the admissions tutors from your personal statement that you are not 100% committed to physiotherapy and therefore your application will not be taken seriously. Also, it will cause you problems writing your personal statement when giving reasons for your desire to have a career in physiotherapy.

If you decide that you would be happy to accept an alternative if your application for physiotherapy is unsuccessful, by all means choose another course, as long as you feel able to justify the choice at interview. However, our advice is to apply only to physiotherapy courses because:

- the way you write the personal statement should demonstrate to the selectors that you are committed to becoming a physiotherapist
- you do not run the risk of feeling obliged to accept a place on a course that, at heart, you do not wish to take. If you are unsuccessful in your initial application for physiotherapy you may be able to gain a place through UCAS Extra or Clearing, if you have accepted no alternative offers.
- the more places you apply to, the more chances you are giving yourself.

Once you have made your final choices, make sure that you have entered the details into the application correctly. More advice on this can be found in *How to Complete Your UCAS Application* (Trotman Education).

> 'When choosing your universities, I found it helpful in my decision making to visit each one. You can get a sense of the university as well as the city or town itself. Open days at universities are so beneficial as the course you are thinking of applying for is explained to you by the department itself. This is the main reason I chose to come to Birmingham to study. The facilities and teaching staff were very impressive and engaging, and their range of course subjects was outstanding. Work placements throughout the study period at Birmingham were impressive thanks to it being a huge, vibrant city with so many differing opportunities. Their employment rates for graduating students was the highest out of my other choices also.'
>
> Jonathan, Birmingham

The UCAS application form

UCAS Hub (previously known as UCAS Track) is UCAS's online applications system, which you can use to register and apply to your university choices. The UCAS application is made up of several important sections. The form is straightforward but it does take time to fill in so do not rush it, as that is when you make mistakes. The sections are as follows:

- **Choices**: your five researched university choices
- **Personal details**: basic information – name, age, title and gender
- **Contact and residency**: address, email, telephone number
- **Nationality**: birthplace and nationality
- Supporting Information: anything universities and providers may need to know to understand what support you might require during your studies
- **English language skills**: to determine whether English is your first language
- **Finance and funding**: details of who is paying your tuition fees
- **Education**: past exam results, information about previous and current schools/colleges, as well as upcoming examinations.
- **Employment**: this is only for paid work, not for any work experience – you should include the employer's name and address
- **Personal statement**: a 4,000-character (including spaces) statement detailing why a university should choose to accept you. Importantly, it should include details of your work experience as the main section. Remember, this is not an essay. Do not use anyone else's words for your personal statement – remember that UCAS has software that will detect this. Check what you have written for accuracy of spelling, punctuation and grammar. Do not be too emphatic – let the content be what will impress an admissions tutor, not your ability to use synonyms (see Chapter 5).
- **Reference**: this is very important. If you are applying through a school, your tutor will write a statement supporting your application and endorsing your potential for the course. Every school has its own guidelines, but in general the reference should comment on your skills, your abilities and your academic results to date, provide the reasons for any poor results and an explanation of what is being done to rectify this, and also a recommendation to the university of you as a student. If you are applying as an independent candidate, you will need to find an academic or professional referee who will follow these guidelines and seek references from other sources to bolster their reference. Referees should read the 'Advisers' section on the website.

Do not rush the application. Take your time and pay attention to the details. Make sure that you have used the correct course and institution codes. Check that you have entered the correct examination boards for your subjects and that all of the dates are accurate. Ensure accuracy throughout the form. Do not miss the deadline, which is usually in the second half of January.

For physiotherapy, the following should also be your guide.

Application checklist

- At least two weeks of NHS work-shadowing?
- Voluntary work?
- Right GCSE subjects and grades?
- Right A level subjects?
- On target for required grades?
- Looked at all the universities' prospectuses?
- Open days?
- Minimum of four physiotherapy choices in the UCAS application?
- Personal statement demonstrates commitment, research, personal qualities, communication skills and manual dexterity?

For more details about UCAS and filling in your application, see *How to Complete Your UCAS Application* (Trotman Education).

Although all information is correct at time of writing, in January 2023 UCAS released its report *Future of Undergraduate Admission* outlining a number of potential reforms to the application process, most notably to the format of the reference and the replacement of the 4,000-character personal statement with a set of questions. Further details are yet to be announced, but the personal statement changes will be introduced no earlier than the 2024 application cycle (2025 entry).

Making your application stand out

When your UCAS application is received by the university it will not be on its own but in a batch of, possibly, several hundred. The selectors will have to consider it, along with the others, in between the demands of their 'real' jobs. If your application is uninteresting, lacking evidence of real commitment to physiotherapy or badly worded, it will be put on the reject pile.

Interviews are an essential part of the UCAS process for physiotherapy. You can be called for interview only on the basis of your UCAS application. The selectors will not know about the things that you have forgotten to say and they can get an impression of you only from what is in the application. We have come across too many good students who never got an interview simply because they did not think about the UCAS application; they relied on the hope that the selectors would somehow see through the words and get an instinctive feeling about them. The following sections will tell you more about what the selectors are looking for and how you can avoid common mistakes. Before looking at how the selectors go about deciding whom to call for interview, however, there are a number of important things that you need to think about.

> 'The best thing about candidates is that they are all different. They are all unique. Therefore our advice is clear; don't write as though you are the same as everyone else. Find the things that are personal to you, your motivations, your values and translate them into your writing. This is our first chance to meet candidates so they need to show their personality. Is the personal statement important? Of course it is. There is a term that we use in application terms: value added. What can this student contribute to the university, the profession and society as a whole. That last point is incredibly important, particularly now as the government changes in the NHS have thrown physiotherapy to the forefront of outreach programmes to promote general health.'
>
> *Admissions tutor*

The personal statement

This is the most important part of your application, as this is where you convince the selectors that you are a serious and suitable candidate. Advice on writing your personal statement is given in the next chapter.

The reference

As well as your results and your personal statement, the selectors will take your reference into account. This is where your head, housemaster or housemistress or head of sixth form writes about what an outstanding person you are – the life and soul of the school; how you are on target for three A grades at A level; and why you will become an outstanding physiotherapist. For him or her to say this, of course, it has to be true.

The referee is expected to be as honest as possible and to try to accurately assess your character and potential. You may believe that you have all of the qualities, both academic and personal, necessary in a physiotherapist, but unless you have demonstrated these to your teachers they will be unable to support your application. Ideally, your efforts to impress them will have begun at the start of the sixth form (or before); you will have become involved in school activities, you will have been working hard at your studies and you will be popular with students and teachers alike. However, it is never too late, and some people mature later than others, so if this does not sound like you, start to make efforts now to impress the people who will contribute to your reference.

As part of the reference your referee will need to predict the grades that you are likely to achieve. If your predicted grades are lower than what is required for your chosen physiotherapy courses it is unlikely that you will be considered. Talk to your teachers and find out whether you are on target for the necessary grades. If not, you need to:

- work harder or more effectively – and make sure that your teachers notice that you are doing so, and/or
- get some extra help either at school or outside, for instance by taking an Easter revision course, and/or
- delay submitting your UCAS application until you have your A level results. If you decide on this option, make sure that you use your gap year wisely (see below).

When to submit the UCAS application

The closing date for receipt of the application by UCAS in 2024 will be 6 p.m. on 31 January.

Late applications are accepted by UCAS but the universities are not obliged to consider them. Because of the pressure on places, it is unlikely that late applications will be considered. Although you can submit your application any time between the beginning of September and the January deadline (remembering to get it to your referee at least two weeks before the deadline so that he or she has time to prepare the reference), most admissions tutors admit that the earlier the application is submitted, the better your chance of being called for interview. Your best bet is to talk to the person who will deal with the application in the summer term of your first year of A levels, and work on your personal statement and choice of universities over the summer holidays so that the application is ready to hand in at the start of the September term.

Deferred entry

Most admissions tutors are happy to consider students who take a gap year, and many encourage it. However, if you are considering this, you need to make sure that you are going to use the time constructively. A year spent watching daytime TV is not going to impress anybody, whereas independent travelling, charity or voluntary work either at home or abroad, work experience or a responsible job will all indicate that you have used the time to develop independence and maturity. Above all, make sure that whatever you do with the year involves regular contact with other people. It is a good idea to check with each individual institution that you are applying to whether they will accept a deferred application. Some advantages of a deferred year are that you can

4 The UCAS application

arrange to be overseas, either travelling or on a work or voluntary placement without the worry of returning for college interviews. Also, it gives you another opportunity during this year to apply for other courses if your first application was unsuccessful.

You can either apply for deferred entry when you submit your UCAS application, in which case you need to outline your plans in your personal statement, or apply in the September following the publication of your A level results. If you expect to achieve your predicted grades and the feedback from your school or college is that you will be given a good reference, you should apply for deferred entry; but if you are advised by your referee that you are unlikely to be considered, you should give yourself more time to demonstrate to your referees that you have what it takes by waiting until you have your A level results.

What happens next?

You can follow the progress of your application using the UCAS online track system, which will show you when your form was sent to the universities and their responses.

The next correspondence you will receive, if you are lucky, is likely to be from the universities, asking you to attend an interview. Do not be alarmed if you do not hear anything soon after UCAS has sent you your statement of entry. Some universities interview on a first-come, first-served basis, while others wait until all applications are in before deciding whom to interview.

If you are unlucky you will receive a message from UCAS telling you that you have been rejected by one or more of the universities. Do not despair; you may hear better news from another of the places that you applied to. Even if you get five rejections, the worst thing that you can do is give up and decide that it is no longer worth working hard. On the contrary, if this does happen, and you are not holding any offers, then you can still use UCAS Extra. This allows you to add another choice of university. If you are unsuccessful and did not achieve the grades required for the universities of your choice then you will be automatically entered for Clearing on the UCAS website. The process of making Clearing applications is discussed on page 84.

5 | Tweak it
The personal statement

Be interesting. That is the takeaway message from this chapter. Speak to any admissions tutor and they will tell you that what they want is to read something that maintains their interest. Keep it factual and make it personal. What they are not looking for is a shopping list of your experiences. Look at everything from the point of view of, 'what has this gained me and how has it inspired me to do this course?'

The personal statement is your opportunity to demonstrate to the selectors that you have not only researched physiotherapy thoroughly, but also have the right personal qualities to succeed as a physiotherapist. There are some universities that do not interview students and therefore they need to see all the information that they are looking for in the personal statement. This chapter will guide you on what you should say and how you should say it.

Why physiotherapy?

A high proportion of UCAS applications contain the sentence: 'From an early age I have wanted to be a physiotherapist because it is the only career that combines my love of science with the chance to work with people.' Not only do admissions tutors get bored with reading this, but it is also clearly untrue; if you think about it, there are many careers that combine science and people, including teaching, pharmacy, dentistry and nursing. However, the basic ideas behind this sentence may well apply to you.

If so, you need to personalise it. You could mention an incident that first got you interested in physiotherapy – a visit to a physiotherapist, a conversation with a family friend or a lecture at school, for instance. You could write about your interest in human biology, or about a biology project that you undertook when you were younger, to illustrate your interest in science, and you could give examples of how you like to work with others. The important thing is to back up your initial interest in physiotherapy with your efforts to investigate the career.

What have you done to investigate physiotherapy?

This is the one part that cannot be stressed highly enough. This is where you describe your work experience (or what you have done instead to investigate physiotherapy if social distancing measures impacted your ability to gain such experience). It is important to demonstrate that you gained something from the work experience and that it has given you an insight into the profession. You should indicate the length of time that you spent at each work placement, what treatments you observed and your impressions of physiotherapy.

You could comment on what aspects of physiotherapy attract you, what you found interesting or something that surprised you. Merely saying where you worked and what you saw is not enough: the selectors want to know what you learnt from the experience. Here is an example of a description of work experience that would not impress the selectors.

> 'I have spent six months volunteering at my local care home. Over this time I have seen various physiotherapy treatments, including ultrasounds, hydrotherapy and massages. I have also enjoyed learning how exercises can help the residents to maintain their mobility. Overall, it has been very interesting and informative.'

The next example would be much more convincing because it is clear that the student was interested in what was happening.

> 'During my six months volunteering at Oak Park care home, I was fortunate enough to shadow their resident physiotherapist. I watched a range of treatments, including ultrasound and exercise in the hydrotherapy pool. At Oak Park, they mainly used hydrotherapy as treatment for the residents with arthritis. It was especially beneficial for them as the warmth of the water allows their muscles to relax, allowing them to exercise as the pain in their joints was eased. As some of the residents are stroke victims, I also got to spend some time with a specialist neurological physiotherapist which was eye-opening. I learned that in these cases the physiotherapist has to physically assist the body in doing things it no longer has the ability to do itself, therefore these treatments are more hands-on and intense. I feel lucky to have had the chance to learn about a different branch of physiotherapy, as it was not an area I had come across before. Seeing first-hand the positive difference physiotherapy can make has only reaffirmed my goal to pursue a career as a physiotherapist.'

With luck, the selectors may pick up on this at interview and ask questions about the methods that the physiotherapists used; the student could then bring in his or her knowledge of ultrasound (having investigated it following the work experience). This student would also gain extra credit with the admissions tutors for having arranged a lengthy work experience placement. Also, what admissions tutors look favourably on would be differing work experience placements, such as working with children or maybe disabled physiotherapy work. The greater the variety of work you have undertaken the more attractive and interesting you are to the interviewer.

Personal qualities

As a physiotherapist you will be working with others throughout your career. To qualify as a physiotherapist you will study alongside maybe 30 others in your year, for three years.

> **TIP!**
>
> The person reading your UCAS application has to decide two things: whether you have the right personal qualities to become a successful physiotherapist, and whether you will cope with and contribute to university life.

To be a successful physiotherapist you need to be able to relate to other people; to survive and enjoy university you need to be able to get on with a wide range of people too. Unlike school life, where many of the activities are organised and arranged by the teachers, almost all of the social activities at university are instigated and organised by the students. For this reason the selectors are looking for people who have the enthusiasm and ability to motivate others and are prepared to give up their own time to arrange sporting, dramatic, musical or social activities.

It is also important to mention manual dexterity. Do you have any particular skills that show this, for example: playing a musical instrument; juggling; origami? Essentially, anything goes provided it shows your dexterous ability. After all, this is a career that involves you using your hands!

Extracurricular activities

How, then, does the person reading your personal statement know whether you have the qualities that they are looking for? They will expect to read about some of the following:

- participation in team events or general teamwork
- involvement in school plays or concerts
- positions of responsibility
- work in the local community
- Duke of Edinburgh Award
- part-time or holiday jobs
- charity work.

The selectors will be aware that some schools offer more in the way of activities and responsibilities than others, and they will make allowances for this. You do not have to have gone on a school expedition to India or to be head girl to be considered, but you need to be able to demonstrate that you have taken the best possible advantage of what is on offer. The selectors will be aware of the type of school or college that you have come from (there is a box on the back of the UCAS application that your referee fills in) and, consequently, of the opportunities that are open to you. What they are looking for is that you have grasped these opportunities. This section should be no longer than a paragraph long. Cover the key points you feel are important; you will have an opportunity to discuss these further at interview.

General tips

- Do not attempt to copy passages from other sources and incorporate them into your personal statement. UCAS uses anti-plagiarism software when checking statements; if you have used material from someone else (including the examples in this book), you will be caught out and your application will be void.
- Do not be tempted to get someone else (a friend, teacher, parent or one of the many internet sites that offer 'help') to write your personal statement. It has to sound like you, which is why it is called a personal statement.
- Although you can apply for up to five institutions or courses, you write only one personal statement, and so it needs to be relevant to all of the courses you are applying for. You will not be able to write a convincing statement if you are applying to a variety of different courses.
- Print off a copy of your personal statement so that you can remind yourself of all the wonderful things you said, should you be called for interview!
- If you are applying for deferred entry, state your reasons for doing so and outline what you intend to do during your gap year. For example, you might be planning to find some relevant work experience in a private practice, and then spend some time overseas volunteering with children.
- Do not be tempted to use overly formal or long-winded English.

5 The personal statement

- Read through a draft of your statement and ask yourself: 'Does it sound like me?' If not, rewrite it.
- Avoid phrases such as 'I was fortunate enough to be able to shadow a physiotherapist ...' when you really mean 'I shadowed a physiotherapist ...' or 'I arranged to shadow a physiotherapist ...'
- Make sure you get someone else to read through it for you, perhaps your teacher or your parent/s. You can become so immersed in the personal statement that you don't see spelling mistakes or grammatical errors. A 'fresh set of eyes' is always best!

First sample personal statement

Physiotherapy is playing an ever more significant role in healthcare worldwide. Having studied biology, geography and food technology at A level, I have gained great insight into how a healthy balanced lifestyle, through nutrition, exercise and health education, has led to increased longevity on a global scale. As healthcare costs rise and greater strain is put on clinics, surgeries and hospitals to provide treatment, I truly believe the future of medicine lies in preventative care, health promotion and rehabilitation; all key aspects of physiotherapy.

Studying biology at A level has allowed me to learn more about human function, including how both the nervous and circulatory system work together to carry out key processes such as respiration and muscle contraction, something that I think will be useful when studying physiotherapy. Through geography, I have seen how demography affects the life expectancy and healthcare demands of different countries, allowing me to discover a range of challenges faced within physiotherapy.

I undertook an e-placement with the NHS Talent Academy, which was my first 'Introduction to Physiotherapy'. Although my interest in sports first drew me towards physiotherapy, this placement opened my eyes to the full breadth of knowledge that physiotherapists require in order to tailor treatment to individual patients across a wide range of different illnesses. I was motivated by the chance to help not only athletes, but patients of all different profiles.

As coronavirus restrictions eased, I secured a placement at Southampton General Hospital. I was shocked to see how quickly an event such as a heart attack and complications during surgery that resulted in two resuscitations could cause such disability to a previously fit and healthy man. Equally, I was amazed in the amputee rehabilitation ward how quickly after surgery physiotherapists could have a patient walking on prosthetics, a process I had assumed would have taken a long time to adapt to.

In contrast to working with humans, I spent a week observing how physiotherapy also benefited animals, including horses and dogs. Further challenges were faced here: physiotherapists relied heavily on their observational skills, since they had no means of communication with the patient other than through the owner. Here I also improved on my communication and organisational skills: contacting patients, making appointments and filing treatment notes.

I have found great satisfaction in volunteering within the community. At Treloar's, a school for disabled children, communication and trust were the main emphasis. Here, I saw how a physiotherapist relied upon the movement of a child's eyes to determine how the child felt, and to find out about their difficulties and view on the treatment they received, since they were unable to communicate verbally. I have also volunteered at Riding for the Disabled and at my local junior school. I have loved getting involved with the children, teaching them new skills including reading, writing and horse riding. Once a bond was formed, the children became more and more trusting, revealing to me their true potential which was really rewarding.

I seek to maintain a healthy and active lifestyle myself, regularly playing lacrosse and tennis at college, and horse riding (where I have competed for my area, both individually and as a team, and also in British Eventing up to BE100 level). I also enjoy cooking and textiles, which I think improves my manual dexterity for the profession. Achieving my Gold Duke of Edinburgh Award has been a highlight: I learnt commitment, leadership and communication skills, which will be vital, as physiotherapy places as much need on a team as well as an individual.

The work experience I have carried out over the past few years has motivated and inspired me to enter an occupation that helps to give a level of independence back to those faced with short-term or terminal illness.

Second sample personal statement

I believe that there are two ways to consider disability: one is to focus on the lack of ability, and the other is to focus on the ability that remains. I grew up with disabled siblings and quickly learned that a disability needn't define a person. Working within boundaries led to unique outcomes and with every challenge disability brought, an opportunity arose.

My sister has Down's syndrome and I used to point out that her condition should be renamed 'Up' syndrome as she was always smiling and enthusiastic. The development of my deaf brother's lip-reading skills showed me the potential people have to overcome the limitations of their disabilities – provided someone is there to help every step of the way. I participated in his rehabilitation and therapy, playing a key role in building up his confidence in speaking.

I was diagnosed with a rare disorder that meant my knees would dislocate as my legs went into flexion. Using the same resilient attitude ingrained in me from childhood, I overcame my movement limitations through seven years of gym training, creating innovative ways to strengthen my body to the point that I could lift weights at a competitive level. My efforts stabilised my joints, happily granting me a completely normal life. So, it is no wonder that I have a passion for fitness and an intense compassion for people with physical problems.

Discovering my true vocation has taken some time. I have travelled the world witnessing poverty and primitive healthcare in many counties. This gave me perspective and an appreciation for the quality of NHS care and the implications a good healthcare system has on society. Having personally received NHS physiotherapy for my condition, I know that without the tenacity with which my care team conducted their investigations, my health and livelihood would have been compromised. My desire to work alongside medical practitioners, with an aim to reduce the compromises society makes with its health, was solidified by these experiences.

For the last eight months I worked at Six Physio, a private physiotherapy network of clinics. My role was administrative support to the ten clinics in London. I learned to embrace the demands of sometimes-difficult clients, treating all with respect, dignity and kindness. I was particularly interested in their Oncology Department. While researching the work of hospitals such as The Royal Marsden, I found the 2017 Macmillan report's piece entitled Physical Activity and Cancer. Evidence of improved quality of life with physiotherapy was outlined including 'moderate improvements in cardiorespiratory fitness and small increases in muscular strength' for cancer patients. The cancer research unit at Kings College aiming to 'develop potential new treatments and prevention strategies for women with breast cancer' is equally inspiring. However, 60% of the 2 million people living in the UK with cancer have unmet physical needs. This statistic furthered my desire to take on the high demand for physio-based cancer treatments in the NHS.

Working under pressure while investigating a problem source is a proficiency I developed while attaining my qualification to become a wine sommelier. Once qualified, I was able to identify a wine's origin from its smell and taste by deconstructing its components. With the high turnover of patients in the NHS, the need for physiotherapists that have a fast-working, investigative mindset is critical. I am determined to combine my analytical skill with the application of university knowledge to help to fulfil this need.

Whether it is a simple rehab exercise to change bad posture or post-cancer strength conditioning, the endurance it takes to stay committed to daily goals is a skill my insight into chronic pain and disability has given me. I have developed a determined outlook when faced with adversity and I hope to be honoured one day with the opportunity to use physiotherapy to empower my patients to look beyond their physical limitations.

Following on from studies carried out as part of *Reimagining UK Admissions*, UCAS has suggested that the personal statement element of the UCAS application will undergo some changes in future. According to the January 2023 report, *Future of Undergraduate Admission*, the personal statement is likely to be replaced by structured questions, with six key areas of questioning being identified so far. It is worth noting that any changes will be introduced no earlier than the 2024 application cycle (for entry onto courses in 2025).

6 | At full stretch
The interview

If the selectors like the picture that the UCAS application has painted of you they may call you for interview. The purpose of the interview is to allow them to see whether this picture is an accurate one and to investigate whether you have a genuine interest in physiotherapy. You must be aware of current events in the profession; this is discussed in Chapter 7. The interviewers will generally ask you three types of question:

1. those designed to relax you so that they can assess your communication skills
2. those designed to investigate your interest in and suitability for physiotherapy
3. those designed to get a clearer picture of your personal qualities.

Sometimes the question will be no harder than 'Why this university?' However, that can catch many out, so make sure you have done even the basic research before your interview.

Questions to get you relaxed

'How was your journey here today?'

The interviewers are not really interested in the details of your travel. Do not be tempted to give them a minute-by-minute account of your bus journey ('... and then we waited for six minutes at the road works on Corporation Street ...'), but also do not simply say 'OK'. Say something like: 'It was fine, thank you. The train journey took about two hours, which gave me the chance to catch up on some reading.' With a bit of luck they will ask you what you read, which gives you the chance to talk about a book, newspaper article or an item in *Frontline*, the magazine of the Chartered Society of Physiotherapy (CSP).

'I am interested to know why you decided to apply to Grantchester.'

Another variation on this might be: 'How did you narrow your choice down to five universities?' The panel will be looking for evidence of research and that your reasons are based on informed judgement.

Probably the best possible answer would start with 'I came to your open day ...', because you can then proceed to tell them why you like their university so much, what impressed you about the course and facilities and how the atmosphere of the place would particularly suit you. Even if you are unable to attend open days, try to arrange a formal or informal visit before you are interviewed so that you can show that you are aware of the environment, both academic and physical, and that you like the place. If you know people who are at the university or on the course, so much the better.

You should also know about the course structure. On pages 18–20 there is an overview of the differences and similarities between courses, and the prospectus will give detailed information. Given the choice between a candidate who is not only going to make a good physiotherapist but clearly wants to come to their institution, and another who may have the right qualities but does not seem to care whether he or she studies there or somewhere else, whom do you think the selectors will choose?

Answers to avoid include the following:

- 'Reputation' (unless you know in detail the areas for which the university is highly regarded).
- 'It's in London, and I don't want to move away from my friends.'
- 'You take a lot of retake students.'
- 'My dad says it is easy to get a place here.'

A good answer could be: 'I came to an open day last summer, which is why I have applied here. I enjoyed the day, and was impressed by the facilities, and by the comments of the students who showed us around because they seemed so enthusiastic about the course. Also, my cousin studied English at the university and I visited her, and got to sample the atmosphere of the town.'

There are variations on this question. The interviewers may ask you what you know about the course, or about the university. In all cases, this is your chance to show the interviewers that you are desperate to come to their university.

> **WARNING!**
>
> Do your homework by reading the prospectus and looking at the website. Although on the surface all physiotherapy courses appear to cover broadly the same subjects, there are big differences in how the courses are delivered and in the opportunities for patient contact, and your interviewers will expect you to know about their course.

Questions about physiotherapy

'Why do you want to be a physiotherapist?'

This is the question that all interviewees expect. Given that the interviewers will be aware that you are expecting the question, they will also expect your answer to be planned carefully. If you look surprised, and say something like 'Um ... well ... I haven't really thought about why ...', you can expect to be rejected. Other answers to avoid are: 'The money'; 'I couldn't get into medicine'; 'I want to help people'; 'I want to work for Arsenal'.

Many students are worried that they will sound insincere when they answer this question. The way to avoid this is to try to bring in reasons that are personal to you, for instance an incident that started your interest (perhaps a visit to a physiotherapist), or an aspect of your work experience that particularly fascinated you. The important thing is to try to express clearly what interested you rather than to generalise your answers. Rather than say 'Physiotherapy combines science, working with people and the chance to have control over your career', which says little about you, tell the interviewers about the way in which your interest progressed. Here is an example of a good answer.

> 'When I was involved with athletics for my club and taking part in events I also volunteered to help with the junior members of the team. From this came the opportunity to be involved with dealing with their injuries firsthand and assisting in their recovery, alongside the team physiotherapist. I always knew that I wanted to be involved with athletics even after my body has given up on me! Therefore, I saw becoming a physiotherapist as a great way to do this. I started taking an active commitment to learning more about physiotherapy by reading relevant materials and also volunteering at my local NHS physiotherapy ward.'

> **WARNING!**
>
> Do not learn this passage and repeat it at your interview. Ensure that your answer is not only personal to you, but also honest.

With luck, the interviewers will pick up on something that you said about work experience and ask you more questions about this. Since 'Why do you want to be a physiotherapist?' is such an obvious question, interviewers often try to find out the information in different ways. Expect questions such as 'When did your interest in physiotherapy start?', 'What was it about your work experience that finally convinced you that physiotherapy was for you?' or 'I see that you spent two weeks with your physiotherapist. Was there anything that surprised you?'

Variations on this question could include 'Was there anything that particularly interested you?', 'Was there anything you found off-putting?' or simply 'Tell me about your work experience'. What these questions really mean is: 'Are you able to show us that you were interested in what was happening during your work experience?' To return to the original question, answering either 'Yes' or 'No' without explanation will not gain you many marks. Similarly, saying 'Yes, I was surprised by the number of patients who seemed very scared' says nothing about your awareness of the physiotherapist's approach to his or her patients.

However, answering 'Yes, I was surprised by the number of patients who seemed very scared. What struck me, however, was the way in which the physiotherapist dealt with each patient as an individual, sometimes being sympathetic, sometimes explaining things in great detail and sometimes using humour to relax them. For instance ...' shows that you were interested enough to be aware of more than the most obvious things.

Sentences that start with 'For example ...' and 'For instance ...' are particularly important, as they allow you to demonstrate your interest. In order to be able to give examples, you should keep a diary of things that you saw during your work experience so that you do not forget. You should read through this before your interview, as if you were revising for an examination.

'I see that you try to keep up to date with developments in physiotherapy. Can you tell me about something that you have read about recently?'

If you are interested in making physiotherapy your career, the selectors will expect you to be interested enough in the subject to want to read about it. Good sources of information are the CSP's website and others (addresses are given in Chapter 11), *Frontline* and the national newspapers. You should get into the habit of looking at a respected newspaper every day to see if there are any medical or physiotherapy-related stories.

Note that the question uses the word 'recently': recent does not mean an article you read two years ago – keep up to date. You could, for instance, say: 'There was a recent report that sportspeople risk injury from wearing air-filled training shoes. There was a survey of basketball players that showed that they were four times more likely to suffer ankle injuries if they were wearing trainers with soles that contained air pockets.'

'During your work experience, you had the chance to discuss physiotherapy with physiotherapists. What do you know about career opportunities and pay for physiotherapists?'

You must make sure that you do some research on career paths by asking questions about this when you meet physiotherapists.

Most physiotherapists work in the NHS, but there are many other options. On pages 7–11 we described many of the types of work undertaken by physiotherapists. Most physiotherapists end up specialising in one or more particular areas – in most cases as a result of an interest that grew during their training. The best answer to a question like this is to describe the career paths of physiotherapists you have met and worked with, as this will allow you to highlight your own work experience.

'What qualities should a physiotherapist possess?'

These have been discussed on page 47. However, do not simply list them. The question has not been asked because the interviewer is puzzled about what these qualities are; it has been asked to give you a chance to show:

- that you are aware of them, and
- that you possess them.

The best way to answer this is to use phrases such as 'During my work experience at the Grantchester Physiotherapy Clinic I was able to observe/talk to the physiotherapist, and I became aware that ...', or 'Communication is very important. For instance, when I was shadowing my physiotherapist, there was a patient who ...' Try always to relate these general questions to your own experiences.

'Physiotherapy requires high levels of physical fitness and manual dexterity. Do you possess these?'

Manual manipulation of a patient's limbs requires a fair degree of fitness and strength, and as a physiotherapist you will need to be able to help to lift and lower patients. If you have trouble picking up a coffee cup without breathing heavily for the next 10 minutes, physiotherapy may not be the best career for you. The interviewers will need to be reassured that you are able to work in a physically demanding environment, and also that you have the manual dexterity necessary to perform sometimes intricate tasks. Try to anticipate this question by preparing an answer that demonstrates that you have these qualities. Sport is always a good indicator of fitness and coordination, but you could also mention situations that you encountered during your work experience, demanding tasks that you perform as part of a weekend job, expeditions that you have been on at school as part of the Duke of Edinburgh's Award, or a hobby such as DIY.

> **WARNING!**
>
> Do not lie about the example you describe. An admissions tutor I talked to recounted the story of an applicant who wrote in the UCAS application that he worked for a local Riding for the Disabled scheme. However, the previous interview had been with someone from the same town who had explained that there was no such scheme in the area, which is why she could not carry on doing this when she moved there. He was found out, and rejected.

Questions to find out what sort of person you are

'What do you do to relax?'

Do not say 'watch TV' or 'go to the pub'. Mention something that involves working or communicating with others, for instance sport or music. Use the question to demonstrate that you possess the qualities required in a physiotherapist. However, do not make your answer so insincere that the interviewers realise that you are trying to impress them. Saying 'I relax most effectively when I go to the local physiotherapy clinic to shadow the physiotherapist' will not convince them.

'How do you cope with stress?'

Physiotherapy can be a stressful occupation. Physiotherapists have to deal with difficult people, those who are scared and those who react badly when in a physiotherapy ward. For many people, physiotherapy can be painful and distressing and patients are not always cooperative, or even aware of why they are receiving treatment. In these circumstances the physiotherapist cannot panic, but must remain calm and rational. The interviewers will want to make a judgement as to whether you will be able to cope with the demands of the job.

Having been through them themselves, it is unlikely that they will regard school examinations as being particularly stressful. Hard work, yes, but not as stressful as training to be a physiotherapist or practising as a physiotherapist. What they are looking for are answers that demonstrate your calmness and composure when dealing with others. You could relate it to your work experience, or your Saturday job. Dealing with a queue of angry and impatient customers demanding to know why their cheeseburgers are not ready can be difficult. Other areas that can provide evidence of stress management are school expeditions, public speaking or positions of responsibility at school or outside.

'I see that you enjoy reading. What is the most recent book that you have read?'

The question might be about the cinema or theatre, but the point of it is the same: to get you talking about something that interests you. Although it may sound obvious, if you have written in your UCAS application that you enjoy reading, make sure that you have actually read something recently. Admissions tutors will be able to tell you stories about interviewees who look at them with absolute amazement when they are asked about books, despite it featuring in the personal statement.

Answers such as 'Well ... I haven't had much time recently, but ... let me see ... I read *Elle* last month, and ... oh yes ... I had to read *Jane Eyre* for my English GCSE' will do your chances no good at all. By all means put down that you like reading, but make sure that you have read an interesting novel in the period leading up to the interview, and be prepared to discuss it.

How to succeed in your interview

You should prepare for an interview as if you are preparing for an examination. This involves revision of your work experience diary so that you can recount details of your time with physiotherapists, revision of the newspaper, website and *Frontline* articles that you have saved, and revision of all of the things that you have mentioned on your personal statement.

> 'Although I was nervous before my interview, I think I was prepared enough to answer all the questions well. I had been advised by a teacher to take my time and think about the question, rather than rush in to an answer, which was good advice. I also had some questions prepared for the end of the interview. I asked about dropout rates and work placements, which I believe showed the interviewer that I was both prepared and serious about the course.'
> Simon, University of Sussex

When you are preparing for your A levels you sit a mock examination so that the real thing does not come as a total surprise; when you are preparing for an interview, have a mock interview so that you can get some feedback on your answers. Your school may be able to help you. If not, independent sixth-form colleges usually provide a mock interview service. Friends of your parents may also be able to help. If possible, video your mock interview so that you are aware of the way you come across in an interview situation. There is a list of practice interview questions overleaf.

Mock interview questions

Questions about you (general)

- Why do you want to be a physiotherapist?
- Why does physiotherapy interest you more than medicine/nursing/radiography?
- What are the ideal qualities that a physiotherapist should possess and do you think you possess those qualities?
- Give me an example of how you cope with stress.
- What have you done to demonstrate your commitment to the community?
- What would you contribute to this university?
- What are your best/worst qualities?
- What was the last novel you read? What did you think of it?
- What was the last play/film you saw? What did you think of it?
- What do you do to relax?
- What is your favourite A level subject?
- What grades do you expect to gain in your A levels?
- What branch of physiotherapy interests you the most and why?
- Why are you taking a gap year?

Questions related to your research into physiotherapy/the university and relevant work experience (example/anecdotal)

- What have you done to investigate physiotherapy?
- Why did you apply to this university?
- Did you come to our open day?
- During your work experience, did anything surprise or shock you?
- Was the physiotherapist you shadowed good at communicating with his/her patients?
- Have you read any articles about physiotherapy recently?
- Why are communication skills important for physiotherapists?
- What have you done that demonstrates your communication skills?
- What have you done that demonstrates your leadership skills?
- What have you done that demonstrates your ability to cope in a stressful situation?
- How did you organise your work experience?
- How does teamwork apply to the role of a physiotherapist?

Questions about physiotherapy (academic)

- Tell me about preventative physiotherapy.
- What is occupational therapy?
- What is repetitive strain injury?
- What is cystic fibrosis/a stroke/arthritis?

- What is hydrotherapy?
- What is ultrasound and how is it used?
- Is exercise always good for you?
- How much do NHS physiotherapists earn?
- What advances can we expect in physiotherapy technology/treatment in the future?
- What precautions need to be taken with patients who are HIV positive?
- What is the role of a physiotherapist in a hospital?
- Why is a knowledge of physics helpful in physiotherapy?
- What are the particular difficulties that animal physiotherapists encounter?

MMIs

There is a growing use of MMIs (Multiple Mini Interviews) now at the application stage. The School of Healthcare Sciences at Cardiff University, for example, uses a series of short and closely-timed interviews in order to get candidates to think on their feet. They provide the following guidance on the purpose and usage of the interview technique:

> 'Interviews help us to determine if you:
>
> - can think on your feet
> - have thought about some of the issues that are important to the profession
> - can critically appraise information
> - can communicate ideas effectively.
>
> 'They also focus on exploring the personal qualities and attributes that are important to your future career development.
>
> 'These interviews allow us to assess information that isn't always readily forthcoming in the application process – they aren't intended to test the amount of prior knowledge you have about the subject or the profession.
>
> *Information taken from www.cardiff.ac.uk/study/undergraduate/courses/course/physiotherapy-bsc, with kind permission from Cardiff University.*

NB: The university does now clarify that if you instead are invited to an online interview, it may not follow the MMI format.

If you are going to attend an MMI then it is a good idea to ask multiple members of staff at your school to ask you different questions and get you to think on your feet.

Sample MMI questions

Station #1:

PROMPT (Read and consider for 2 minutes):

A friend tells you that her dad has been battling alcoholism for years and it has put a strain on the family. They are thinking they will have to leave their studies and go home to help out in the family as it is all too much right now. How do you counsel your friend?

RESPOND: (Speak max. 8 minutes)

Station #2:

PROMPT (Read and consider for 2 minutes):

What do you think are the major sorts of problems facing a person with a long-term health problem, such as arthritis?

RESPOND: (Speak max. 8 minutes)

Station #3:

PROMPT (Read and consider for 2 minutes):

Imagine you are on a committee able to recommend only one of two new treatments to be made available through the NHS. The treatments are: an artificial heart for babies born with heart defects, or a permanent replacement hip for people with severe arthritis. Both treatments are permanent, i.e. never need repeating, and are of equal cost. On what grounds would you make your arguments?

RESPOND: (Speak max. 8 minutes)

Station #4:

PROMPT (Read and consider for 2 minutes):

Can you think of something you'd like to invent?

RESPOND: (Speak max. 8 minutes)

Station #5:

PROMPT (Read and consider for 2 minutes):

Give us an example of something about which you used to hold strong opinions, but have had to change your mind. What made you change? What do you think now?

RESPOND: (Speak max. 8 minutes)

Appearance and body language

Appearance and body language are important. The impression you create can be very influential. Remember that if the interviewers cannot picture you as a physiotherapist in future years they are unlikely to offer you a place.

Body language

- Maintain eye contact with the interviewers.
- Direct most of what you are saying to the person who asked you the question, but occasionally look around at the others on the panel.
- Sit up straight, but adopt a position that you feel comfortable in.
- Do not wave your hands around too much, but do not keep them gripped together to stop them moving. Fold them across your lap, or rest them on the arms of the chair.

Speech

- Talk slowly and clearly.
- Do not use slang.
- Avoid saying 'erm …', 'you know' or 'sort of'.
- Say 'hello' at the start of the interview, and 'thank you' and 'goodbye' at the end.

Dress and appearance

- Wear clothes that show you have made an effort for the interview.
- You do not have to wear a business suit, but a jacket and tie or a skirt and shirt/blouse are appropriate.
- Make sure that you are clean and tidy.
- If appropriate, shave before the interview (but avoid overpowering aftershave).
- Clean your nails and shoes.
- Wash your hair.
- Avoid (visible) piercings, earrings, jeans and trainers.

At the end of the interview

You may be given the opportunity to ask a question at the end of the interview. Bear in mind that the interviews are carefully timed, and that your attempts to impress the panel with 'clever' questions may do quite the opposite. The golden rule is: ask a question only if you are genuinely interested in the answer (which, of course, you were unable to find during your careful reading of the prospectus).

Questions to avoid

- What is the structure of the first year of the course?
- Will I be able to live in a hall of residence?
- When will I first have contact with patients?

As well as being boring questions, the answers to these will be available in the prospectus. You have obviously not done any serious research.

Questions you could ask

- 'Are my A levels enough of a foundation before starting this course or could you recommend something else I should review before starting?' Proactive.
- 'Do you think I should try to get more work experience before the start of the course?' Again, an indication of your keenness.
- 'Earlier, I couldn't answer the question you asked me on ultrasound. What is the answer?' Something that you genuinely might want to know.
- 'How soon will you let me know if I have been successful or not?' Something you really want to know.

> **REMEMBER!**
>
> If in doubt, do not ask a question. End by saying 'All of my questions have been answered by the prospectus and the students who showed me around the university. Thank you very much for an interesting day.' Smile, shake hands (if appropriate – if you are being interviewed by a panel of five, who are all sitting at the other end of a long table, then do not!) and say goodbye.

Structuring the interview

The selectors will have a set of questions that they may ask, designed to assess your suitability and commitment. If you answer 'Yes' or 'No' to most questions, or reply only in monosyllables, they will fire more and more questions at you. If, however, your answers are longer and also contain statements that interest them, they are more likely to pick up on these and you are, effectively, directing the interview. If you are asked questions that you have prepared for there will be less time for the interviewers to ask you questions that might be more difficult to answer.

For example, at the end of your answer to a question about work experience, you might say '… and the physiotherapist was able to explain the effect of new technology on physiotherapy.' The interviewer may then say: 'I see. Can you tell me about how technology is changing physiotherapy?' You can then embark on an answer about ultrasound, for instance. At the end of your explanation you could finish with: '… of course, ultrasound treatment is often used in conjunction with infrared radiation treatment.' You might then be asked about situations where this might happen, and so on.

Of course, this does not always work, but you would be very unlucky not to have at least one of these 'signposts' followed that you placed in front of the interviewers.

How you are selected

During the interview the panel will be assessing you in various categories. Whether or not the interview appears to be structured, the interviewers will be following careful guidelines so that they can compare candidates from different interview sessions. Some panels adopt a conversational style, whereas others are more formal. The scoring system will vary from place to place but, in general, you will be assessed in the following categories:

- reason for your choice of university
- academic ability
- motivation for physiotherapy
- awareness of physiotherapy issues
- personal qualities
- communication skills.

You are likely to be scored in each category, and the university will have a minimum mark that you will have to gain if you are to be made an offer. If you are below this score, but close to it, you may be put on an official or unofficial waiting list. If this happens you may be considered in August, should there be places available.

If you are offered a place you will receive a letter from the university telling you what you need to achieve in your A levels. This is called a conditional offer. Post-A level students who have achieved the necessary grades will be given unconditional offers. If you are unlucky, all you will get is an email from UCAS saying that you have been rejected. If this happens it is not necessarily the end of the road that leads you to a career in physiotherapy.

If you are rejected by all of your choices, you can enter the UCAS Extra scheme, which allows you to contact other universities. If you still are without a place when the A level results are released in August, you will be eligible to apply for vacant places through Clearing.

When UCAS has received replies from all of your choices it will send you a Statement of Offers. You will then have about a month to make up your mind about where you want to go. If you have only one offer you will have little choice but to accept it. If you have more than one you will have to accept one as your firm choice and another (usually a lower offer) as your insurance choice. If the place where you really want to study makes a lower offer than one of your other choices, do not be tempted to choose the lower offer as your insurance choice, since you will be obliged to go to the university that you have put as your firm choice if you achieve the grades. Even if you narrowly miss the grade, you may still be accepted by your first choice. If you decide that you do not want to go there, once the results are issued, you will have to withdraw from the UCAS system for that year.

> 'It's so important that prospective students understand what physiotherapists do. They have to comprehend the depth of the job. Prospective students need to show compassion and motivation. When people are in pain it's not easy to get them moving. You have to show empathy rather than sympathy.'
>
> *Admissions Tutor*

7 | Do you know your gluteus maximus from your articulatio cubiti?
Current issues

This chapter explains the most relevant current issues in physiotherapy. This should be used as a reference point for your interview but not as your only source of information. You should make sure that you read newspapers and journals (such as *Frontline*) to get ideas on other current issues and not just rely on those listed here. Your success at interview will depend on your ability to converse fluently on up-to-date topics. You do not have to be an expert in your field – that is what the interviewers are – but you do need to have tried to understand the profession that you wish to follow. If that comes as a surprise, this is not the right career for you!

The NHS Long Term Plan

With the NHS turning 70 years old in 2019, the NHS Long Term Plan, first published in January 2019, aimed to ensure its future success. The plan sets out a range of aims to make sure everyone gets the best start in life, to deliver world-class care for major health problems and the support of people into their older years. There was to be improved funding of 3.4% over the following five years, compared to 2.2% over the previous five years. The plan was put into effect after consulting patients' groups, professional bodies and frontline NHS leaders.

In relation to physiotherapy, the plan saw the physiotherapy workforce as key to successfully delivering the changes, with prevention and rehabilitation at the forefront. Furthermore, there is support for increasing the number of personnel to deal with primary and community care, along with the increase of funding.

This launch, by NHS England's Simon Stevens, has been seen as a major breakthrough for physiotherapy and the treatment of patients. A promise to create many more first-contact physiotherapist roles and wider access to rehabilitation across a range of conditions sees a number of positive references to the profession.

Professor Karen Middleton, chief executive of the CSP, said:

> 'It marks the clear shift towards providing services in the community that we have long called for, and places an emphasis on prevention.
>
> 'It explicitly sets out the integral role physiotherapy staff, including first contact physiotherapists, will make in delivering this transformation.
>
> 'Crucially, it also sets out targets on rehabilitation across a number of conditions, which will serve to focus minds when designing and commissioning services.
>
> 'We will go through the detail in the coming days and it is already obvious that there remain unanswered questions about workforce and social care funding, among other issues. These must be addressed if we are to achieve the success the plan aspires to.
>
> 'But as a blueprint for how the NHS should proceed with physiotherapy playing a crucial role, there is a lot to like in this plan.'

Information taken from the CSP (www.csp.org.uk), with kind permission from the CSP.

The points listed below highlight the key implications for physiotherapy as a result of the NHS England Long Term Plan.

Overall

- Prevention and rehabilitation are key themes throughout the plan.
- The physiotherapy workforce is identified as essential to successfully delivering the plan.
- There is support for expanding the physiotherapy workforce in primary and community care.
- There is commitment to increasing the funding of both primary and community services as a proportion of the overall health budget.
- Digital infrastructure will be deployed to improve data collection, access to services, personal health records and to support self-care.
- There is a commitment to invest in physiotherapy workforce development. However, specific commitments on CPD and career development are still focused on nurses and doctors.
- There is no mention at all of the unregistered physio/Allied Health Professions (AHP) workforce.

Primary Care

- The first contact physio (FCP) model will be endorsed as part of a new vision for integrated primary and community services. It will be implemented beyond the existing pilots.
- FCPs will be part of the 'GP Forward View' workforce targets for the first time.
- Physiotherapists will be part of the primary care workforce in rapid response teams.
- Digital technology will enable GP appointments to be bookable via NHS 111.
- Primary care networks will have a role in the early diagnosis of Chronic Obstructive Pulmonary Disease (a similar approach to the frailty index in General Practice).

Community Rehabilitation

- Community rehabilitation is highlighted as an area for significant development.
- There is a proposal for integrated community hubs, with physiotherapy as part of multi-disciplinary teams.
- There is a specific commitment to expand pulmonary, cardio and stroke rehabilitation.
- Needs assessments for stroke and cancer patients will include rehabilitation after discharge.

Information taken from the CSP (www.csp.org.uk), with kind permission from the CSP.

The NHS England Long Term Plan contains many encouraging ideas and directives for all those involved in and around physiotherapy. Patients will be able to book convenient appointments directly with physios and other expert health professionals at a local practice, without the need to wait for a referral or travel to a specialist clinic.

Professor Stephen Powis, NHS National Medical Director, said: 'More physios based in community GP surgeries means people have more choice and can get the treatment they need without waiting weeks to make what can be a long journey to hospital for a short appointment, and is a great example of how the NHS Long Term Plan will increasingly deliver more care options closer to home over the coming years.'

Concussion

Despite being in the spotlight for a few years already, the 2022 Football World Cup in Qatar once again drew attention to how concussion appears to be overlooked in elite football after Iran's goalkeeper was allowed to play on despite suffering a head injury that took ten minutes to treat. Physiotherapists can continue to play a key role in educating sportsmen and women about concussion.

Clinical update: Concussion

According to a report in the CSP's *Frontline* magazine, minor head trauma isn't just a sports injury:

> 'Physios in all specialisms can help to spot undiagnosed concussion that needs treatment.
>
> 'Concussion is a minor traumatic brain injury caused by a blow to the head or violent head movement, such as in a traffic collision. Although there is often no outward damage, and the patient usually stays conscious, the jolt may briefly disrupt electrical activity in the brain.
>
> 'It's more common among sports players, young men, older people and those who are homeless or have mental health problems. Children and teenagers take longer to recover and are more likely to suffer long-term damage. Having concussion more than once increases the risk of long-term damage.
>
> 'Among sports players, evidence suggests that women are more likely to have concussion, and that the risk may be related to the menstrual cycle, with experts noting that sportswomen often recover slower from concussion than sportsmen.
>
> 'Anyone suffering a head injury should be monitored over several days as bleeding inside the skull is not immediately obvious.
>
> 'In sport, there are new laws around head injuries. Any head injury should be treated as serious and the player be immediately removed from the field of play and not allowed to return during the match. They should then be properly medically assessed. There should be a minimum period of one week's rest and then the Graduated Return To Play programme is applied, once the symptoms have stopped. This is a minimum of one week and they need to be carefully monitored by medical staff and physiotherapists.'

Information taken from the CSP (www.csp.org.uk), with kind permission from the CSP.

The role of a physiotherapist

All physiotherapists in any field may find themselves in the situation of saving a life. Any bump on the head could cause minor brain trauma and this could lead to bigger problems in the future. Physiotherapists can pick up on signs or indicators that a patient might be suffering more than they let on, or even perhaps more than they know. A good example in physiotherapy is that of vestibular rehabilitation. This is used in the treatment of a loss of balance but if concussion is involved, the patient may be suffering from other after effects that require looking at and possible treatment.

Symptoms to look out for are: drowsiness, dizziness, nausea, headache or pressure in the head, loss of memory, difficulty in understanding or communicating, sensitivity to light or noise. If they are encountering severe neck pain, deteriorating consciousness, increasing confusion or irritability, severe headache, repeated vomiting, unusual behaviour, convulsions, problems with seeing or hearing or weakness or tingling in arms or legs, then you should seek immediate medical attention.

Technology in physiotherapy

Enter the words 'physiotherapy' and 'news' into an internet search engine and most of the links that you get are to news stories about new forms of treatment. Although the basic techniques used in physiotherapy have been around for a long time – physical manipulation, repetition of exercises and other forms of manual therapy – technology plays an increasingly important role.

Probably the most widely used application of technology within physiotherapy is ultrasound. Ultrasound treatment utilises high-frequency (up to 3MHz – too high for the human ear to hear) sound waves. Ultrasound is used extensively in medicine for diagnosis, either to form images in order to see what is happening inside the body (for instance, scans that show a foetus inside the womb) or to measure blood flow.

Whenever ultrasound waves pass from one tissue to another, a small percentage of the beam is reflected back, and these reflected sound waves are used to create a picture, or to measure the speed at which blood is flowing (using something called the Doppler effect). Ultrasound can also be used therapeutically; that is, for treatment. It has been used to accelerate tissue repair and to relieve pain since the 1950s. It is used to treat a variety of conditions, such as sports injuries, sprains, tendonitis, arthritis and ulcers, and to relieve the pain associated with, for instance, phantom limbs in amputees. The sound waves penetrate deep into the body and, although the biological effects are not completely understood, it is likely that the vibration caused by the sound waves produces a combination of heating (thermal effects) and stimulation of tissue and blood vessels (mechanical effects). Ultrasound is usually given at the end of a course of treatment, following other forms of manual therapy.

Ultrasound equipment is relatively cheap to buy (less than £2,000 for an ultrasound machine) and is easy to use. The drawbacks of the extensive use of ultrasound in physiotherapy are that there is little conclusive clinical evidence that it is effective and that there is a possible risk of tissue damage if the power settings on individual machines are not calibrated accurately.

Another treatment that utilises sound waves, extracorporeal shockwave therapy (ESWT), has been introduced into physiotherapy clinics. ESWT was brought to a wider audience in 2004 when Sachin Tendulkar, the Indian cricketer, received shockwave therapy to treat tennis elbow that had failed to respond to conventional physiotherapy. Developed from the devices that generate pulses of sound waves to destroy kidney stones, ESWT devices produce pulses of high-pressure sound that travel through the skin. Soft tissue and bone that are subjected to these pulses of high-pressure energy heal back stronger. Tennis elbow results from calcification of a tendon and is usually treated with mechanical exercise or steroid injection (which risks weakening the tendon still further), but new treatments are also being developed.

There are instances of robots being used in physiotherapy. This does not mean that next time you require physiotherapy you will be treated by R2-D2, Bender or Kryton. The effective rehabilitation of patients with cerebral palsy, or following a stroke or other brain injuries, requires repetitive movement exercises and controllable resistance to motion. In one such treatment the patient is coupled to a robot joystick that guides him or her through a series of movements. The robot can be programmed to vary the scope of the movement, to increase or decrease the resistance, or to help the patient to complete the movements. To increase interest levels for the patient, the movements can be integrated into a 'game' on a screen in front of the patient. In this way tens of thousands of therapeutic movements can be completed over the course of a few weeks – far more than the physiotherapist could manage, and more than the patient is likely to be able to accomplish alone.

One of the biggest and most comprehensive advances in physiotherapy is The Performance Matrix (TPM). This is a collection of analytical software that identifies the weak points and high-risk areas of your movement, such as your back or joints. TPM involves performing roughly 15 movement tests to identify these points, the results of which are calculated immediately. TPM is used to aid rehabilitation and recovery, as well as injury prevention. For this reason, it has proven popular not just with people who have sustained an injury, but also for professional athletes looking to maximise their performance.

Though still a relatively young technology, virtual reality (VR) is providing a lot of exciting opportunities for all sorts of different medical professionals. One of the biggest advantages of this is the immersiveness of VR, which enables people in remote areas to exercise as if they were in a class full of people. It also helps monitor their movements and keep them on the right track. Additionally, VR can be used to make the exercises much more fun and even something people enjoy, making patients more likely to stick with their regimen. You can expect to see VR become commonplace in the next few years.

Another technological advance for physiotherapy is the creation of apps that are designed to help people address their physiotherapy issues independently. For example, there is one app that allows you to locate over 100 trigger points in over 70 muscles, and another that helps you to understand prevention of future medical needs; one that corrects spinal posture; and another that measures range of motion. In this modern age, millions of people are wearing fitness tracker watches and wristbands to measure their steps, heart rate and general levels of activity. This information can be used to calculate and track a range of other things, such as how many calories you've burned.

Equally, the rise of social media is having an effect on the profession; specifically Twitter. Physios are now able to tweet exercise tips to a wider audience, ensuring those with low mobility, or simply those with a busy lifestyle, are keeping on top of their fitness.

Mental health

Research has been undertaken that demonstrates that around one in five people with osteoarthritis has suffered from depression or anxiety at one time or another. Also, a third of people who have suffered a stroke have endured a depressive episode. If physiotherapists fail to recognise symptoms while working with recovering patients, then the results could be fatal. Valuing the physical health of people with mental health issues is essential to patient rehabilitation and continuing progress. Patients undertaking around 120 minutes a week of physical activity are around 30% less likely to develop depression or anxiety in the future.

An ageing population

> 'In mid-2020 there were 1.7 million people aged 85 years and over, making up 2.5% of the UK population. By mid-2045, this is projected to have nearly doubled to 3.1 million, representing 4.3% of the total UK population. There are projected to be many more people at older ages by 2045, in part because of the baby boomers from the 1960s now being aged around 80 years as well as general increases in life expectancy.'
>
> Information taken from the Office for National Statistics (www.ons.gov.uk).
Contains public sector information licensed under the
Open Government Licence v3.0.

At present, there is a strain on physiotherapy services, which have to deal with the effects of ageing and mobility among the elderly. Physiotherapy services therefore need to focus on facilitating independence among the elderly so that they are not dependent on the health services or care facilities to cope with normal life. Physiotherapy should also enable those still of working age to continue working, thus reducing the need for early retirement. A factsheet on musculoskeletal disorders (MSDs) published by the CSP highlights that MSDs are the most common physiotherapy problem treated among the workforce and are therefore a priority to be addressed in order to prevent further problems down the line.

Prescribing more activity for older people is part of a more proactive approach by physiotherapists to prevent a loss of mobility and independence.

A 2015 article in the *Guardian* newspaper states that 'Starting an exercise regime in your 70s or 80s may sound unusual. But for a growing number of older people it could help them hold on to their independence for longer, and reduce the pressure on families, carers and the health and social care system.' The article goes on to explain in more detail how this can be achieved. '"There is a lot of evidence that physical activity and exercise are valuable however old you are, and that frail, older people gain the most benefit," says Louise McGregor, vice-chair of the Agile professional network for physiotherapists working with older people. "You are really never too old. We now have a lot more people who live into their 100s and they can still benefit from the right type of exercise."'

Another area where physiotherapy could have a lasting benefit is with people with dementia. Physiotherapists can have a key role in assessing a patient's needs and giving high-quality care. Louise McGregor says that creative, adaptable strategies are important for such patients, as while an elderly person with dementia would benefit from a physiotherapy or exercise programme, they may well forget to follow it.

Obesity

Obesity is one of the biggest health challenges that we face in this country. It is an issue that the government is now actively trying to combat, as 28% of adults in the UK are currently obese, and a further 36.2% are overweight. Statistics from the Department of Health's Foresight report, which looked into ways of responding to rising obesity in the UK, indicated that if the trend continues, then by 2050, nine in 10 adults will be overweight. While this is roughly still the case, recent modelling has shown that by 2030, 41% to 48% of men and 38% to 43% of women will be obese. The annual cost to the NHS is estimated to be £6.5 billion;

and the social annual cost (i.e. cost to society) in the UK is around £58 billion. These sums have jumped significantly in recent years, partly due to the Covid-19 pandemic.

As we have already discussed, prevention is just as important as cure. In August 2016 a government 'childhood obesity strategy' was published highlighting the dangers of high sugar intake. In 2018, sugar levies on soft drinks were introduced, as well as guidance on calorie-reduction programmes. This was preceded by schemes such as the healthy-eating Change4Life movement, nowadays named Healthier Families. The CSP recommends that an adult should exercise five times a week at moderate intensity for roughly 30 minutes. If that is not physically possible, i.e. you have time constraints that do not allow a concentrated period of exercise, then manage your time effectively and split the 30 minutes into shorter sessions at different intervals throughout the day. It may sound obvious, but this will have a positive effect on your health if continued over a long period of time.

The campaign is designed to show people that increased levels of physical activity can prevent, or help to control, more than 20 medical conditions, most notably obesity, osteoarthritis, heart disease, type 2 diabetes and other conditions affecting well-being such as depression. If nothing else, the release of endorphins through increased levels of activity will have a positive effect on productivity and output during a working day. It is a complete endorsement of the adage 'healthy body, healthy mind'.

Childhood obesity

Childhood obesity and excess weight are significant health issues for children and their families as there can be serious implications for a child's physical and mental health, which can continue into adulthood. The number of children with an unhealthy and potentially dangerous weight is a national public health concern. Healthcare professionals play an important role in supporting families to take action. Working alongside physiotherapists and other public health teams, they can also influence the population as a whole by delivering system approaches to tackle excess weight, and help reduce drivers of excess calorie intake and sedentary lifestyles.

The statistics are compelling, and the pandemic-related lockdowns in 2020 and 2021 worsened further young people's participation in physical activity. Sport England found that fewer than half now participate in at least 60 minutes of physical activity per day, while almost half do not even achieve 30 minutes. A 2022 study by Swansea University also found children in Wales to be among the least active in the world. The website www.kidshealth.org has great recommendations on how children can improve their health with simple and effective ideas.

A government report on childhood obesity stated that: 'Low levels of physical activity, and increased sedentary behaviours among children and young people, exacerbate the problems of poor diet and nutrition. Boys are more likely than girls to meet the recommended levels, as are children from the most affluent families when compared with the least affluent families.'

Parkinson's disease

Parkinson's is a progressive neurological condition characterised by motor and non-motor problems. The main changes arise from brain dysfunction through reduced production of chemical messengers, particularly the neurotransmitter dopamine.

Drug therapy and deep brain stimulation can provide partial relief of symptoms but many people require additional support from allied health interventions including physiotherapy, which was rated as a top priority by respondents to the membership survey conducted by the charity Parkinson's UK.

Physiotherapy involvement is supported by a growing evidence base of high-quality research, which is informing best practice guidelines. Short-term patient benefits in a range of physical and quality of life measures have been identified through systematic reviews.

Physiotherapy assessment and management focuses on improving physical capacity and quality of movement in daily life through walking and transfer training, balance and falls education, and practice of manual activities (e.g. reaching and grasping). Other issues, e.g. pain, well-being, respiratory function and support networks, may need attention.

The two main areas of Parkinson's-specific physiotherapy intervention relate to exercise and movement strategy training. During the earlier stages, physiotherapists emphasise education and self-management, encouraging use of leisure and third-sector programmes that promote general fitness and inclusion in community activity. Physiotherapy-specific exercise can offset the effects of Parkinson's to minimise deterioration in strength, endurance, flexibility and balance.

As the condition progresses, physiotherapists teach and apply movement strategies to overcome difficulty in generating automatic movement and thought, including developing strategies to compensate for loss of function, using external (auditory, tactile, visual and sensory) or internal (mental rehearsal and visualisation) cues, dual task training, self-instruction and improving attention span.

Physiotherapy is essential in the multidisciplinary management of people with Parkinson's. Advice and education offered in the early stages maintains general fitness, minimises deterioration and promotes self-management. In the later stages, physiotherapy can improve gait, balance, transfers, manual activities and reduce the falls risk.

Information taken from the CSP (www.csp.org.uk), with kind permission from the CSP.

Repetitive strain injury

Repetitive strain injury (RSI) is an increasingly common complaint among computer users. As the name suggests, the condition is caused by repetition of certain movements, usually associated with computer keyboard use. However, RSI is not confined to computer users and has been diagnosed in many people whose jobs involve manual labour or machine operation. Prevalence has been especially noted within the armed forces and among construction, textile processing and other processing workers. The condition can also occur when the person's posture is inappropriate to the task that he or she is undertaking. It is recognised as one of the most common workplace injuries, with the Trades Union Congress (TUC) reporting that 500,000 UK workers have reported an RSI, resulting in a total loss of 5.4 million working days a year.

RSI manifests itself as pain, mostly when the task that caused it is being carried out, but often at other times as well. It usually affects the neck, shoulders, elbows, wrists or hands. RSI is also known by other names, including WRMSD (work-related musculoskeletal disorder), WRULD (work-related upper limb disorder), CTD (cumulative trauma disorder) and OOS (occupational overuse syndrome). The term RSI actually encompasses a number of different conditions, most commonly carpal tunnel syndrome. 'Carpal' comes from the Greek word *karpos*, which means wrist. The joint in the wrist is surrounded by fibrous tissue and there is a small gap between this tissue and the bone, through which a nerve (the median nerve) passes. The nerve then splits to serve the fingers and thumb. Repetitive movement of the wrist can cause swelling of the tissue in the wrist, putting pressure on the median nerve. Symptoms include numbness and tingling in the fingers and thumb, followed by pain. The condition can usually be cured by a combination of physiotherapy and rest.

Not everyone believes that RSI actually exists. Carpal tunnel syndrome certainly does, and can be caused by obesity, arthritis, diabetes and pregnancy, but some people are sceptical as to whether repetitive movement is a cause. A report in the *British Medical Journal* on research done at Manchester University cast some doubts on RSI. The research indicated that the majority of those who suffered from arm or wrist pain (105 people in a survey involving 1,200 volunteers) were also the most dissatisfied with their jobs and suffered from high stress levels. In other words, the pain could be due to psychological or stress factors rather than simply the physical aspects of their jobs.

Rehabilitation of stroke patients

A stroke occurs when a blood clot blocks a blood vessel in the brain, causing brain cells in the area to die. If treatment is not given immediately, further cells in the surrounding areas also die. The functions that were controlled by those brain cells (such as speech, memory or movement) are then affected, depending on the area of the brain where the blood vessels were blocked. The severity of the stroke can vary from patient to patient. The effects may be very minor (and temporary) or they may lead to paralysis or death.

The main types of rehabilitation are:

- physical therapy – to improve mechanical skills such as walking, use of the hands, or balance
- occupational therapy – to re-learn the skills that are required for everyday life such as eating, dressing and looking after oneself
- speech therapy – to re-learn how to communicate effectively.

Physiotherapy for stroke patients must begin as early as possible following the stroke in order to be effective. Improvement is slow and recovery is difficult six months after the stroke. However, paralysed muscles must not be treated too early or they may be damaged permanently.

Research carried out at the University of Texas and reported in *New Scientist* found that rats and monkeys that had received small brain injuries to cause paralysis of a limb suffered further injury if treatment was started immediately. The researchers surmised that glutamate, a neurotransmitter that is released during movement, was the probable cause, since, in large concentrations, it acts as a toxin. Brain damage appeared to multiply its effects. Research is now being carried out to find drugs that will block the effects of glutamate.

> *'Some of these drugs block a receptor group to glutamate called N-methyl-D-aspartate (NMDA). Investigative NMDA antagonists include remacemide, memantine, riluzole, and budipine. Budipine is of particular interest. It not only blocks NMDA, but it increases levels of two enzymes involved in the production of dopamine.'*
>
> Information taken from www.truthinlabeling.org, with kind permission from the Truth in Labelling Campaign.

The expertise of the physiotherapist is vital in assessing when (and in what form) treatment should start. At the start of the treatment, the physiotherapist will prepare muscles for the more intensive treatments that will follow, and will work on enabling the patient to support his or her own weight if leg muscles are affected. The later stages of physiotherapy may involve compensation for permanently damaged muscles through the introduction of aids such as walking frames. The physiotherapist may work alongside occupational therapists, speech therapists, carers and psychologists to try to prepare the patient for a return to 'normal' life.

Exercise referral schemes

Exercise Referral Schemes are designed to promote physical activity for people who have an existing health condition and are physically inactive. They are used to help patients suffering from a wide range of problems, including:

- coronary heart disease
- diabetes
- hypertension
- mental health problems, including depression
- musculoskeletal problems, e.g. chronic lower-back pain
- obesity
- problems caused by falls.

Self-referral schemes

In 2016, it was reported that a new vision of primary care in England where physiotherapists work alongside GPs as well as other health professionals had been successfully introduced in some parts of the country. NHS Suffolk was providing physiotherapy as the first point of contact in 27 of its sites with promising results: a 30% reduction of patients suffering from musculoskeletal (MSK) issues on their GPs' caseloads. Also, a 40% reduction in patients needing knee and hip replacements has been reported.

With schemes such as these patient needs would be met earlier, and GPs would be able to concentrate on aspects of care only they can provide. Also, allowing patients to self-refer to a physiotherapist would free up more GP appointments and also improve patient satisfaction levels.

Stand up for your health

On average reports say that British people sit for 8.9 hours every day. Many sit for much more than that. Public Health England has issued guidance designed for employers to help them mobilise their staff to increase productivity because in turn this will improve the health of the workforce. They highlight certain findings that point to an increase in high blood pressure, obesity and type 2 diabetes among workers who spend most of their day sat down.

They recommend that all workers should get between two and four hours of standing and light walking per day; that people check their movements on a regular basis and seek physiotherapy where necessary; balance sitting and standing work and where necessary, encourage employers to equip the workplace with sit-stand desks and also employers should promote the message of a healthy work/life balance.

The role of the physio becomes especially important as the increase in activity under this scheme will mean that some people experience musculoskeletal problems. Not only will physios be responsible for the treatment of these injuries but also there is an emphasis on the profession circulating guidance on good practice and exercise techniques in order to minimise the numbers of problem cases.

This is not a new initiative and tends to be highlighted annually, certainly over the past few years. However, current research highlights the developing issue and the links with more serious illnesses, which is once again raising the profile of the need for change.

Physiotherapists given prescribing powers

There are two types of prescribing for physiotherapists:

1. **Supplementary prescribing** is the use of a written clinical management plan (CMP) to prescribe agreed medicines in partnership with a doctor. The CMP can include any licensed or unlicensed medicines and all controlled drugs.
2. **Independent prescribing** is the use of individual clinical reasoning and professional judgement to determine the nature and extent of any medicines to be used in the management of diagnosed and undiagnosed conditions. Independent prescribers may prescribe any licensed medicine from the British National Formulary, within national and local guidelines, for any condition within their area of competence within the overarching framework of human movement, performance and function.

Phil Gray, Chief Executive of the CSP, is quoted as saying, 'This is a landmark moment that will lead to patients receiving faster, more effective treatment for their condition. Physiotherapists being able to independently prescribe – for the first time anywhere in the world – will remove bureaucracy, free up time for doctors and save money for the NHS.'

Brexit and the NHS

By the middle of 2022, the NHS in England was short of 12,000 hospital doctors and more than 50,000 nurses and midwives. It is estimated that a further 475,000 jobs will remain unfilled in health and a further 490,000 in social care by the early part of the next decade. Brexit is blamed by many for the high numbers of staff vacancies, as fewer doctors and nurses are coming to the UK to work for the NHS from EU countries.

Since Brexit, EU citizens are only able to access NHS services if they have a 'pre-settled status'. This means that they must be able to prove that they were living lawfully in the UK on or before 31 December 2020. The deadline for the EU Settlement Scheme has now passed.

If migrating to the UK from the EU for the first time, EU nationals will now pay the 'immigration health surcharge' as part of their visa application – as is the case for nationals of non-EU countries. This is a pre-determined fee according to the number of years of the visa and provides residents (including international students) with access to NHS services. It forms a mandatory part of the visa process. Anybody visiting the UK from an EU or non-EU country for less than six months will not receive a Biometric Residence Permit or pay the immigration health surcharge and is therefore advised to take out health insurance to cover the potential cost of medical care.

Alternative therapies

Physiotherapists are becoming increasingly interested in utilising so-called 'alternative therapies' alongside traditional techniques, such as:

- acupuncture
- Alexander technique
- aromatherapy
- chiropractic medicine
- massage
- reflex therapy.

Acupuncture

Acupuncture originated over 3,000 years ago in China. The practitioner inserts thin needles into the body at designated places in order to help alleviate or cure problems. Nowadays, this may also involve the use of small electric currents. It is thought that the needles stimulate the body's nervous system into producing its own painkilling substances. The safe delivery of acupuncture is monitored by the Acupuncture Association of Chartered Physiotherapists (AACP), a clinical interest group of the CSP.

Alexander technique

The Alexander technique is a method of releasing unwanted muscular tension throughout the body by making the patient aware of balance, posture and coordination while performing everyday actions. It is particularly associated with the performing arts.

Aromatherapy

Aromatherapy uses essential oils that are derived from plants and flowers. The oils are either vaporised and inhaled, or applied directly to the body – often in conjunction with massage.

Chiropractic medicine

Chiropractic medicine aims to address the improper alignment of the vertebrae in the spine, which, it is believed, causes a number of physical disorders. Re-alignment is achieved by manipulation.

Massage

Massage is the manipulation of the soft parts of the body. Physiotherapists with a particular interest can do postgraduate training in many different types of massage. The CSP has a special interest group: Chartered Physiotherapists Interested in Massage and Soft Tissue Therapies (CPMaSTT).

Reflex therapy

Reflex therapy deals with problems within the body by targeting related points on, for example, the feet, hands or head. Reflex therapy can be arranged by consulting a chartered physiotherapist who is a member of the Association of Chartered Physiotherapists in Reflex Therapy (ACPIRT), a clinical interest group of the CSP.

8 | Massaging the results
Results day

The A level results will arrive at your school on the third Thursday in August. IB results will be available at the beginning of July and the Scottish Higher results are released in early August. The universities will have received them a few days earlier. You must make sure that you go into school on the day the results are published. Do not wait for the results slip to be posted to you. Get your teachers to tell you the news as soon as possible – once they are able to, of course! If you need to act to secure a place you may have to do so quickly. The following paragraphs take you through the steps necessary to use the UCAS Extra, Clearing and Clearing Plus systems. They also explain what to do if your grades are disappointing.

The university admissions departments are well organised and efficient, but they are staffed by human beings. If there were extenuating circumstances that could have affected your exam performance and which were brought to their notice in June, it is a good idea to ask them to review the relevant letters shortly before the exam results are published.

If you previously received a conditional offer and your grades equal or exceed that offer, congratulations! You can relax and wait for your chosen university to send you joining instructions.

> A word of warning: you cannot assume that grades of AAC satisfy an ABB offer. This is especially true if the C grade is in biology. Always check with your chosen university.

What to do if you have no offer

If all of the universities that you applied to reject you, you are then eligible to enter a scheme called UCAS Extra. This allows you to apply to other universities, either for physiotherapy or for other courses. You will automatically be sent details by UCAS.

UCAS Extra starts in March. If UCAS Extra does not provide you with an offer, then you are eligible for Clearing from July through to September. These days, very few applicants get into university through Clearing. Very few universities have spare places in August and, of those that do, most will choose to allow applicants who hold a conditional offer to slip a grade rather than dust off a reserve list of those they interviewed but did not make an offer to. Still less are they likely to consider applicants who appear out of the blue, however high their grades. That said, it is likely that every summer one or two universities will have enough unfilled places to consider a Clearing-style application.

In order to help students to find these fewer places, UCAS has recently created Clearing Plus. This tool is designed for students who are either applying to university for the first time through Clearing, or for those who were unsuccessful in their original applications. The service seeks to 'matchmake' students with courses that interest them and for which they meet the entry requirements.

If you hold, say, AAB but were rejected when you applied through UCAS, you need to let the universities know that you are out there. The best way to do this is by email. If you live nearby you can always deliver a letter in person, talk to the office staff and hope that your application will stand out from the rest.

Below you will find a sample email. Do not copy it word for word! Do not forget that your UCAS referee may be able to help you. Try to persuade him or her to ring the admissions officers on your behalf – your referee will find it easier to get through than you will. If your head teacher is unable or unwilling to ring, then he or she should at least email a note in support of your application. It is best if both emails arrive at the university at the same time.

From: Jo Carter
To: mdwhyte@grantchester.ac.uk
Subject: Physiotherapy places

Dear Miss Whyte
UCAS No. 15-123456-8

I have just received my A level results, which were: Biology A, Chemistry C, English C. I also have an A grade in AS English Language. You may remember that I applied to Grantchester but was rejected after interview/was rejected without an interview. I am still very keen to study physiotherapy at Grantchester and hope that you will consider me for any places that may now be available. My head teacher supports my application and is emailing you a reference. Should you wish to contact him, the details are:

> Mr S. Honry, tel: 0123 456 7891, email: s.honry@secondary school.ac.uk. I can be contacted at the above email address and could attend an interview at short notice.
>
> Jo Carter

If you are applying to a university that was not one of your original choices and therefore have never seen your UCAS application, ask your head to email or send a copy of your application. Although, in general, it is best to persuade the university to invite you to send the UCAS application to them.

If, despite your best efforts, you are unsuccessful, consider applying again (see page 86). The alternative is to use the Clearing system to obtain a place on a degree course related to physiotherapy, and then apply for physiotherapy again after you graduate (see page 84).

What to do if you hold an offer but miss the grades

If you have only narrowly missed the required grades (this includes the AAC grade case described on page 83) it is important that you and your referee email the university to put your case before you are rejected. Another sample email follows below.

> From: Jo Carter
> To: mdwhyte@grantchester.ac.uk
> Subject: A level results
>
> Dear Miss Whyte
> UCAS No. 15-123456-8
>
> I have just received my A level results, which were: Biology A, Chemistry B, English C. I hold a conditional offer from Grantchester of ABB and I realise that my grades fall below that offer. Nevertheless, I am still determined to study physiotherapy and I hope you will be able to find a place for me this year. I would like to remind you that at the time of the exams I was recovering from glandular fever. A medical certificate was sent to you in June by my head teacher.
>
> My head teacher supports my application and is emailing you a reference. Should you wish to contact him, the details are: Mr S. Honry, tel: 0123 456 7891, email: s.honry@secondaryschool.ac.uk. I can be contacted at the above email address and could attend an interview at short notice.
>
> Jo Carter

Retaking your A levels

Universities' grade requirements for retake candidates are often higher than for first-timers. You should contact the universities to find out what they require from retake students. Many A levels can be retaken, but a student can re-sit only in June, which poses problems of its own. The timescale for your retakes will depend on:

- the grades you obtained first time
- the examination board through which you studied.

If you simply need to improve one subject by one or two grades and can retake the exam on the same syllabus, then a short retake course between January and June is the logical option. However, you do need to consider whether it is realistic for you to re-start study, having not studied the subject for seven months. You also need to consider whether spending a full year on your retakes would give universities more confidence that you will achieve the required grades. The school or college where you will sit the retakes will be able to advise you.

If, on the other hand, your grades were DDE you probably need to spend another year on your retakes.

Independent sixth-form colleges provide specialist advice and teaching for students considering A level retakes. Interviews to discuss this are free and carry no obligation to enrol on a course, so it is worth taking the time to talk to their staff before you embark on A level retakes.

It is worthwhile bearing in mind that students who are now retaking are going to be compared not only with first-time applicants but also with first-time applicants from a new academic system and that may have an effect on decisions.

Re-applying to university

The choice of universities for your UCAS application will be narrower than it was the first time round. Do not apply to universities that discourage retakers unless there really are special, extenuating circumstances to explain your disappointing grades. The following are examples of excuses that would not be regarded by admissions tutors as extenuating circumstances.

- 'I was revising on my dad's yacht and my files got soaked when I accidentally dropped them in the sea.'
- 'I left my bag on the bus the week before the exams, and all of my notes were in it, so I couldn't do any revision.'
- 'We moved house a month before the exams and a removal man trod on my notes, so I couldn't revise properly from them.'

8 Results day

Some reasons are acceptable to even the most fanatical opponents of retake candidates:

- your own illness
- the death or serious illness of a very close relative.

Please note, an extenuating circumstance application is not a different application. The circumstances are really the responsibility of your referee to explain.

These are just guidelines, and the only sure way to find out if a university will accept you is to write and ask. A typical email is set out at the end of this chapter. Do not follow it word for word and do take the time to write to several universities before you make your final choice.

Notice that the format of your email should be:

- opening paragraph
- your exam results: set out clearly, with no omissions
- any extenuating circumstances: a brief statement
- your retake plan: including the timescale
- a request for help and advice
- closing paragraph.

Make sure that your email is brief, clear and well presented. Even if you go to this trouble, the pressure on universities in the autumn is such that you may receive no more than a standard reply to the effect that, if you apply, your application will be considered. Apart from the care needed in making your choice of universities, the rest of the application procedure is as described in the first part of this book.

From: Jo Carter
To: mdwhyte@grantchester.ac.uk
Subject: Application for physiotherapy

Dear Miss Whyte
Last year's UCAS No. 15-123456-8

I am writing to ask your advice because I am about to complete my UCAS application and would very much like to apply to Grantchester. You may remember that I applied to you last year and received an offer of ABB/was rejected after interview/was rejected without an interview. I have just received my A level results, which were: Biology B, Chemistry C, History D. I was aged 16 years and seven months at the time of taking these exams.

I plan to retake Chemistry in June after a 17-week course in the period from January to June, and History over a year. If necessary,

I will also retake Biology in June. I am confident that I can push these subjects up to ABB grades overall.

What worries me is that I have heard that some universities do not consider retake candidates even when the exams were taken under the age of 18 and relatively high grades were obtained. I am very keen not to waste anyone's time by applying to departments that will reject me purely because I am retaking.

I am very keen to study at Grantchester, and would be extremely grateful for any advice that you can give me.

Jo Carter

9 | The fifth metatarsal
Non-standard applications

So far, this book has been concerned with the 'standard' applicant: the UK resident who is studying at least two science subjects at A level or Scottish Highers, International Baccalaureate, Irish Leaving Certificate and BTEC courses and who is applying from school or who is retaking immediately after disappointing results. This chapter outlines the application process for 'non-standard' applicants.

The main non-standard categories are as follows.

Students who have not studied science A levels

If you decide that you would like to study physiotherapy after having already started on a combination of A levels that does not fit the subject requirements for entry to university, you have three choices.

1. You can spend an extra year studying science A levels at a sixth-form college that offers one-year A level courses. You should discuss your particular circumstances with prospective colleges in order to select suitable courses. You need to be aware that only very able students can cover A level Chemistry and Biology in a single year with good results.
2. You can follow a Foundation course at a university that will then allow you to study a related degree course afterwards. For details of Foundation courses you should contact universities.
3. You can enrol on an Access course which is recognised by the universities you wish to apply to. Each university will have different policies about Access courses – you should contact the physiotherapy departments directly.

International students

The competition for the few places available to international students is fierce, and you would be wise to discuss your application informally with the university before submitting it. In general, overseas applicants will find it difficult to gain a place unless they can offer qualifications that are recognised by the universities, such as A levels or the International Baccalaureate (IB). There are, however, bridging qualifications purposely designed for international students that can qualify students for entry into physiotherapy courses, such as the NCUK International Foundation Year in Science.

Information about qualifications can be obtained from British Council offices, British embassies and the universities that offer physiotherapy courses. Overseas students are liable for the full cost of tuition. For physiotherapy the fees vary greatly depending on the university. They can range from £14,000 to £32,000 per year. The UCAS website has a section for international students that describes in detail the application process and deadlines.

English language qualifications

In order to begin a university degree in this country, you are required to have an accredited English language qualification if you are an international student. This is because it is essential that you are able to understand the course and what is being taught to you throughout your studies.

You should aim to achieve at least IELTS (International English Language Testing System) 6.5 to 7.0 in order to begin a university course, and certainly no less than 6.5 in each band. Most universities will set the boundary higher, commonly at 7.0 now, in order to discourage some applications. If you would like further information on IELTS, please visit www.ielts.org.

While IELTS is the most commonly requested English language certificate by universities in the UK, there are a wide range of other English language tests now available, and since the pandemic, UK universities have become more flexible on the certificates they will accept. Other examples of language certificates that will be considered include PTE Academic, TOEFL, LanguageCert, Skills for English and Duolingo. Nevertheless, it remains important to check with your chosen universities that they will accept a certain English language certificate before booking and paying for the test.

Visa requirements

If you require a visa to be in the UK and your course is longer than six months, which physiotherapy courses invariably are, then you will need to apply for a Student Visa. In order to do this, the university you are accepted by will request from you various pieces of information, including your education transcripts and passport. They will produce a Confirmation of Acceptance of Studies (CAS) letter for you once you have given them all the information and paid a specific deposit; you will take the CAS letter to the UK embassy in your country in order to obtain a visa for studying. Do not delay in this process as obtaining a visa can take time, which varies from country to country.

Mature students

Physiotherapy courses are popular with older students, and the universities tend to have a flexible and encouraging approach to students over the age of 21.

Nowadays, more than half of the physiotherapy student cohort is mature students. Work experience is key, as it points to you being a strong candidate and having researched the course properly.

Graduates

A 2.i degree (or higher) along with at least a grade B in A level Biology is normally required for graduates applying for physiotherapy. Most universities ask graduates to take a year out between the final year of their first degree course and the start of the physiotherapy course in order to get work experience. This allows them to demonstrate that they are serious about a career in physiotherapy.

Applicants with no suitable academic qualifications

Candidates are likely to be asked to sit at least two A levels, one of which will be Biology, and to achieve B grades or higher. There are also some Access courses that can lead to an offer of a place to study physiotherapy; applicants should liaise with universities to confirm suitability.

The main difficulty facing those coming late to the idea of studying physiotherapy is that they rarely have a scientific background. They face the daunting task of studying science A levels and need very careful counselling before they embark on what will, inevitably, be quite a tough programme. Independent sixth-form colleges provide this counselling as part of their normal interview procedure.

Access courses

A proportion of colleges of further education offer Access courses suitable for physiotherapy. One well-known example is the course at the College of West Anglia in King's Lynn. Primarily (but not exclusively) aimed at health professionals, they offer a full-time, one-year course in Access to Science and Nursing. It should be noted there are also other providers.

The course that you take might be Access to Science, to Health Studies, to Physiotherapy or to Medical Sciences, but you must cover cardiovascular, pulmonary and skeletal muscle physiology at level 3. Some universities will ask for biology or human biology. You should contact the specific university to find out exactly which Access course it recognises.

You should contact the university admissions tutors or look on the university websites for advice. There is a strong case for suggesting that those people getting in to universities are the ones who put in the work beforehand by talking to the universities. If you have a question, ask it – you will get an answer that you can then base your decision on.

Physiotherapy degree apprenticeships

A degree-standard apprenticeship in physiotherapy is a new entry route into the profession. To be considered for a degree apprenticeship, you will first need to apply for an apprentice position with a healthcare provider; vacancies can be found on the NHS Jobs website and Find an Apprenticeship website. The scheme is primarily a work-based programme, developing the skills and behaviour a student will need to become a physiotherapist. An end-point assessment (EPA) will need to be passed in order to complete the course.

Once you've successfully completed a programme approved by the HCPC, you will then be eligible to apply for registration with the HCPC. Once registered as a practitioner, you'll be required to retain your name on the register by keeping your knowledge and skills up to date through engaging in continuing professional development (CPD) and paying an annual retention fee.

9 Non-standard applications

Students with disabilities and special educational needs

Universities welcome applications from students who have physical or other disabilities or special educational needs, and they have well established support systems in place to provide assistance and special facilities. The services offered can help with a wide range of disabilities, including sensory (visual/hearing) impairment, mental health difficulties, mobility impairment, dexterity impairment, Asperger's syndrome, or other autistic spectrum disorders or chronic medical conditions (e.g. dyslexia or dyspraxia). In all cases you should contact the universities directly before you apply to explain your particular needs and requirements. They will be able to give you information on how they can help you. The website www.disabilityrightsuk.org contains useful links and information.

10 | Make no bones about it
Fees and funding

The following sections explain who pays what in respect of university tuition fees and give you some ideas of where you may find help in funding your studies.

Fees

UK students

Universities are allowed to charge UK students up to £9,250 a year for tuition fees. If you are a student resident in England or Wales you will pay up to £9,250 to study in England, Scotland or Northern Ireland, and up to £9,000 to study in Wales. If you are a student resident in Scotland you won't be liable for tuition fees if you study at a Scottish university, however, you will pay up to £9,250 if you study in England or Northern Ireland, and up to £9,000 if you study in Wales. If you are a student resident in Northern Ireland you will pay up to £9,250 if you study in England or Scotland, up to £9,000 if you study in Wales, but you will pay only £4,710 if you study in Northern Ireland. You should refer to the websites of the specific universities to find out what they intend to charge, and also to the UCAS website, using the course search facility.

International students

EU and non-EU international students now pay the same fees, unless EU candidates hold 'pre-settled status' and are also considered domestic by the university fees assessment. Universities can set their own tariffs for international students. Costs can be found at the universities' individual websites.

Bursaries, sponsorship and grants

NHS bursaries

Home students in England might be eligible to apply for an NHS Learning Support Fund of £5,000 per academic year.

In Wales, students may receive a non-means-tested NHS grant, currently around £1,000 per year, and are eligible for a means-tested NHS bursary to help with day-to-day living costs. All new and prospective students are eligible to apply, and students who are awarded these bursaries can also apply for student loans.

If you've been living in Northern Ireland for the last three years, you can apply for an income-assessed bursary to assist with living costs for health professional degrees there.

At the time of writing, there are no NHS bursaries available for students studying allied health courses in Scotland. While domestic undergraduates can continue to follow the usual student finance processes, mature students already holding a degree may be able to apply for a student loan to cover the first two years of their study.

Contact details for awarding bodies

England
NHS Learning Support Fund
Email: nhsbsa.learningsupportfind@nhsbsa.nhs.uk
Website: www.nhsbsa.nhs.uk/Students.aspx

Wales
NHS Wales Student Awards Services
Email: abm.sas@wales.nhs.uk
Website: www.nwsspstudentfinance.wales.nhs.uk/home

Scotland
Student Awards Agency Scotland
Website: www.saas.gov.uk

Northern Ireland
Student Finance NI
Website: www.studentfinanceni.co.uk

Sponsorship

Sponsorship is also sometimes available from prospective future employers; the armed forces are particularly well known to support students through their training. If you wish to apply for sponsorship from a specific sports club or national body – and bear in mind that some of them will not advertise such schemes – then it is often best to get in touch personally in writing, stating your aims and career aspirations and the course onto which you have been accepted to study.

Maintenance loans

You will still need to find money to pay for your rent, bills, books, food, drink and any hobbies or interests. All money available to Home students for living expenses will be provided as a maintenance loan, to be paid back once students start earning over a particular threshold, which varies according to their home region: £25,000 or more for students from England, £27,295 or more for students from Wales, £25,375 or more for students from Scotland, and £20,195 or more for students from Northern Ireland (all figures correct at time of writing). For further details, please refer to www.gov.uk/student-finance.

Universities charging tuition fees of £9,250 must provide financial support for students from disadvantaged backgrounds. You can find out about this at:

- www.ucas.com/undergraduate/student-life/getting-student-support/undergraduate-student-support
- www.gov.uk/student-finance.

Work while you study

The first people to check with about working while you study are the universities themselves, as some have a policy that you cannot pursue any paid employment while studying this course; but most will merely point out the time commitment involved in the work experience you will be doing as part of your course. That is certainly something to bear in mind as it will be draining in both time and energy for you.

Of course, it is understandable that you may need to find part-time work alongside your course in order to supplement your living and maintenance costs, but just make sure that it does not become a primary emphasis. This is not a course that can be approached half-heartedly and you must make sure that the majority of your spare time is spent pursuing the ultimate end goal.

11 | Exercise the mind
Useful information and further resources

You are advised to check the UCAS Handbook or website for information on courses and universities before applying.

Universities offering physiotherapy degrees

University of Bedfordshire
Tel: 01234 400400
Website: www.beds.ac.uk

University College Birmingham
Tel: 0121 604 1000
Website: www.ucb.ac.uk

University of Birmingham
Tel: 0121 414 3344
Website: www.birmingham.ac.uk

University of Bolton
Tel: 01204 900600
Website: www.bolton.ac.uk

Bournemouth University
Tel: 01202 524111
Website: www.bournemouth.ac.uk

University of Bradford
Tel: 01274 232323
Website: www.bradford.ac.uk

University of Brighton
Tel: 01273 600900
Website: www.brighton.ac.uk

Bristol, University of the West of England
Tel: 0117 965 6261
Website: www.uwe.ac.uk

Brunel University
Tel: 01895 274000
Website: www.brunel.ac.uk

Canterbury Christ Church University
Tel: 01227 928000
Website: www.canterbury.ac.uk

Cardiff University
Tel: 029 2087 4000
Website: www.cardiff.ac.uk

University of Central Lancashire
Tel: 01772 201201
Website: www.uclan.ac.uk

University of Chichester
Tel: 01243 816000
Website: www.chi.ac.uk

Coventry University
Tel: 024 7765 7688
Website: www.coventry.ac.uk

University of Cumbria
Tel: 01228 616234 (Carlisle)
Website: www.cumbria.ac.uk

University of East Anglia
Tel: 01603 456161
Website: www.uea.ac.uk

University of East London
Tel: 020 8223 3000
Website: www.uel.ac.uk

University of Essex
Tel: 01206 873333
Website: www.essex.ac.uk

Glasgow Caledonian University
Tel: 0141 331 3000
Website: www.gcu.ac.uk

University of Gloucestershire
Tel: 01242 714700
Website: www.glos.ac.uk

Glyndŵr University
Tel: 01978 290666
Website: www.glyndwr.ac.uk

11   Useful information and further resources

University of Hertfordshire
Tel: 01707 284000
Website: www.herts.ac.uk

University of Huddersfield
Tel: 01484 422288
Website: www.hud.ac.uk

University of Hull
Tel: 01482 346311
Website: www.hull.ac.uk

Keele University
Tel: 01782 734010
Website: www.keele.ac.uk

King's College London
Tel: 020 7836 5454
Website: www.kcl.ac.uk

Leeds Beckett University
Tel: 0113 812 0000
Website: www.leedsbeckett.ac.uk

University of Leicester
Tel: 0116 252 2522
Website: www.le.ac.uk

University of Liverpool
Tel: 0151 794 5927
Website: www.liv.ac.uk

London South Bank University
Tel: 020 7815 7815
Website: www.lsbu.ac.uk

Manchester Metropolitan University
Tel: 0161 247 6969
Website: www.mmu.ac.uk

Newman University Birmingham
Tel: 0121 476 1181
Website: www.newman.ac.uk

Northumbria University
Tel: 0191 406 0901
Website: www.northumbria.ac.uk

University of Nottingham
Tel: 0115 951 5151
Website: www.nottingham.ac.uk

Oxford Brookes University
Tel: 01865 741111
Website: www.brookes.ac.uk

Plymouth University
Tel: 01752 600600
Website: www.plymouth.ac.uk

Plymouth Marjon University
Tel: 01752 636700
Website: www.marjon.ac.uk

Queen Margaret University, Edinburgh
Tel: 0131 474 0000
Website: www.qmu.ac.uk

Robert Gordon University, Aberdeen
Tel: 01224 262000
Website: www.rgu.ac.uk

University of Salford
Tel: 0161 295 0000
Website: www.salford.ac.uk

Sheffield Hallam University
Tel: 0114 225 5555
Website: www.shu.ac.uk

South Bank University, London
Tel: 020 7815 7815
Website: www.lsbu.ac.uk

University of Southampton
Tel: 023 8059 5000
Website: www.southampton.ac.uk

University of South Wales
Tel: 03455 767778
Website: www.southwales.ac.uk

St George's, University of London
Tel: 020 8672 9944
Website: www.sgul.ac.uk

St Mary's Twickenham
Tel: 020 8240 4000
Website: www.stmarys.ac.uk

University of Suffolk
Tel: 01473 338833
Website: www.uos.ac.uk

11 Useful information and further resources

University of Sunderland
Tel: 0191 515 3000
Website: www.sunderland.ac.uk

Teesside University
Tel: 01642 218121
Website: www.tees.ac.uk

University of Ulster
Tel: 028 7012 3456
Website: www.ulster.ac.uk

University of Winchester
Tel: 01962 841515
Website: www.winchester.ac.uk

University of Wolverhampton
Tel: 01902 321000
Website: www.wlv.ac.uk

University of Worcester
Tel: 01905 855000
Website: www.worcester.ac.uk

York St John University
Tel: 01904 624624
Website: www.yorksj.ac.uk

Useful resources

Chartered Society of Physiotherapy

An essential starting point is the CSP's website (www.csp.org.uk). It carries detailed information about careers in physiotherapy and recognised courses. The CSP also produces many useful booklets about physiotherapy. It can be contacted at:

Chartered Society of Physiotherapy
10 Furnival Street
London EC4A 1AB
Tel: 020 7306 6666

The CSP publishes a magazine, *Frontline*, aimed at practising physiotherapists. The magazine contains articles of interest and is a useful way of keeping up to date with current issues and new developments. There is also a large jobs section – a good way to make contact with physiotherapy practices if you are looking for work experience.

Other societies

Irish Society of Chartered Physiotherapists
Royal College of Surgeons
St Stephen's Green
Dublin 2
D02 H903
Ireland
Tel: +353 1 402 2148
Website: www.iscp.ie

Royal College of Occupational Therapists
106–14 Borough High Street
London SE1 1LB
Tel: 020 3141 4600
Website: www.rcot.co.uk

Royal College of Podiatry
2nd Floor, Quartz House
207 Providence Square
Mill Street
London SE1 2EW
Tel: 020 7234 8620
Website: www.rcpod.org.uk

World Federation of Occupational Therapists
Website: www.wfot.org

UCAS

For information on university applications contact UCAS (www.ucas.com). The UCAS website has a search facility that will enable you to check the latest entrance requirements for all universities that offer physiotherapy courses. Application materials can be obtained from:

UCAS
Rosehill
New Barn Lane
Cheltenham GL52 3LZ

Other useful addresses

Department for Economy (Northern Ireland)
Netherleigh
Massey Avenue
Belfast BT4 2JP
Tel: 028 9052 9900
Website: www.economy-ni.gov.uk

11 Useful information and further resources

NHS (England) Student Bursaries
Tel: 0300 330 1345
Website: www.nhsbsa.nhs.uk/nhs-bursary-students

Student Awards Agency Scotland
Saughton House
Broomhouse Drive
Edinburgh EH11 3UT
Website: www.saas.gov.uk

Student Awards Services (NHS Wales)
Floor 4
Companies House
Crown Way
Cardiff CF14 3UB
Tel: 029 2090 3700
Website: www.nwsspstudentfinance.wales.nhs.uk/home

Useful websites

Examination boards

www.aqa.org.uk
www.ets.org/toefl
www.ielts.org
www.ocr.org.uk
http://qualifications.pearson.com
www.wjec.co.uk

Online physiotherapy information

www.evidence.nhs.uk
www.lifemark.ca
www.naidex.co.uk
www.thephysiotherapysite.co.uk

University league tables

www.theguardian.com/education/universityguide

Work experience

www.prospects.ac.uk

Fees and funding

www.studentfinanceni.co.uk
www.studentfinancewales.co.uk
www.ucas.com/undergraduate/student-life/getting-student-support/undergraduate-student-support
www.gov.uk/education/funding-and-finance-for-students

Further reading

Books on careers/university applications

How to Complete Your UCAS Application, Duncan Chamberlain and UCAS, MPW Guides/Trotman Education

University Degree Course Offers: The essential guide to winning your place at university, Brian Heap, Trotman Education

Books on physiotherapy

There are numerous textbooks covering all aspects of physiotherapy. Most of these are aimed at undergraduates or physiotherapy professionals. The following will give A level (or the equivalent) students an overview of what studying physiotherapy would entail:

A Practical Guide to Sports Injuries, Malcolm T.F. Read, Butterworth-Heinemann

Principles and Practice of Physical Therapy, William E. Arnould-Taylor, Stanley Thornes

12 | Don't be bone idle
Glossary

CCG	clinical commissioning group
CfWI	Centre for Workforce Intelligence
CPD	continuing professional development
CSP	The Chartered Society of Physiotherapy
CTD	cumulative trauma disorder
ESWT	extracorporeal shockwave therapy
Frontline	CSP magazine
Gait re-education	learning to walk with a normal pattern again
HCPC	Health & Care Professions Council
HESA	Higher Education Statistics Agency
HPAT	Health Professions Admission Test (Ireland)
Hydrotherapy	using water in treating pain relief and illness
Infrared and ultraviolet radiation	used to warm damaged muscles and speed up healing
IPE	inter-professional education
MCSP	Member of the Chartered Society of Physiotherapy
MDT	multidisciplinary team
NHS	National Health Service
OOS	occupational overuse syndrome
PBL	problem-based learning
PBPL	practice-based professional learning
Personal statement	part of the UCAS application (4,000 characters with spaces), aimed at persuading universities to accept your application
RSI	repetitive strain injury
SRP	State Registered Physiotherapist
Tennis elbow	calcification of a tendon
UCAS	The Universities and Colleges Admissions Service

Ultrasound	using sound waves to break down scar tissue and reduce inflammation
WRMSD	work-related musculoskeletal disorder
WRULD	work-related upper limb disorder

Postscript

If you have any comments or questions arising out of this book, we and the staff of MPW would be very happy to answer them. You can contact us at the addresses below.

Good luck with your applications!
James Griffith

MPW (London)
90–92 Queen's Gate
London SW7 5AB
Tel: 020 7835 1355
Email: london@mpw.ac.uk

MPW (Cambridge)
3–4 Brookside
Cambridge CB2 1JE
Tel: 01223 350158
Email: cambridge@mpw.ac.uk

MPW (Birmingham)
16–18 Greenfield Crescent
Edgbaston
Birmingham B15 3AU
Tel: 0121 454 9637
Email: birmingham@mpw.ac.uk

Notes

Notes

Have you seen the rest of the Getting into series?

Written by experts in a clear and concise format, these guides go beyond the official publications to give you practical advice on how to secure a place on the course of your choice.

trotman

Helping you get the career you want

Order today from
www.trotman.co.uk/GettingInto